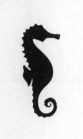

Jacki Sorensen's
AEROBIC

LIFESTYLE BOOK

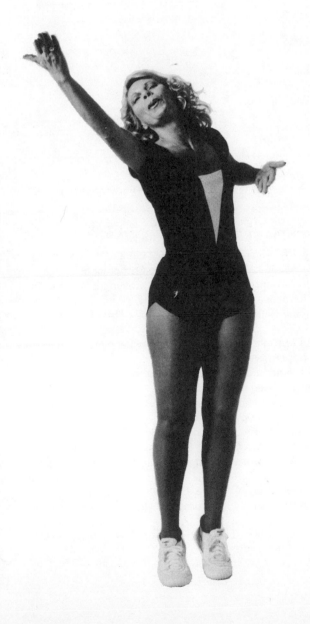

By Jacki Sorensen

with Bill Bruns

POSEIDON PRESS • NEW YORK

10 9 8 7 6 5 4 3 2 1

Library of Congress Cataloging in Publication Data
Sorensen, Jacki.
    Jacki Sorensen's Aerobic lifestyle book.
    1. Aerobic dancing.   2. Aerobic exercises.
3. Diet.   4. Physical fitness.   I. Bruns, Bill.   II. Title.
III. Title: Aerobic lifestyle book.
RA781.15.S68   1983   613.7   83-2231
ISBN 0-671-45616-4

All photographs by Gary Bernstein, with the following exceptions:
    pp. 143–157, photographs by Glen A. Clark of William E. Estabrook Photography; p. 191, photograph by Michael Hart.

The author is grateful for permission to reprint the following song lyrics:

(p. 14, below) *Up Where We Belong* by Will Jennings, Buffy Sainte-Marie and Jack Nitzsche. Copyright © 1982 by Famous Music Corporation and Ensign Music Corporation.

(p. 14, above, and p. 198) *No Time at All* and *Corner of the Sky*. Copyright © 1972 by Stephen Schwartz. All publishing performance and exploitation rights for the world owned exclusively by Jobete Music Co., Inc., and Belwin Mills Publishing Corp. Used with permission. All rights reserved.

(p. 84) *Downhill Stuff* by John Denver. Copyright © 1978, 1979, Cherry Lane Music Publishing Co., Inc. All rights reserved. Used by permission.

(p. 87) *On the Robert E. Lee* by Neil Diamond and Gilbert Becaud. © 1980 Stonebridge Music and EMA-Suisse. All rights reserved. Used by permission.

(p. 200) *Riders to the Stars* by Barry Manilow / Adrienne Anderson / Kamakazi Music / Angela Music, Inc. Administered by Townsway Music. Copyright 1976.

(p. 201) *I'm on My Way* by Alan Jay Lerner and Frederick Loewe. Copyright © 1951 by Alan Jay Lerner & Frederick Loewe; copyright renewed, Chappell & Co., Inc., owner of publication and allied rights throughout the world. International copyright secured. All rights reserved. Used by permission.

(p. 203) *Smile Smile Smile* by Hugo Peretti, Luigi Creatore, George David Weiss. © 1972, 1973 The EMP Company and the Herald Square Music Company. Used by permission. All rights reserved.

(p. 204) *I Want to Live* by John Denver. Copyright © 1977, 1978, Cherry Lane Music Publishing Co., Inc. All rights reserved. Used by permission.

(p. 205) *Jacki's Theme: There's No Stopping Us* by Sister Sledge. Copyright © 1981 by Aerobic Dancing, Inc.

Dedicated to my husband, Neil

With special thanks to my friend
Bill Bruns, who made this book do-able . . .
one word at a time.

APPLAUSE AND A HUG FOR:

Janis "JJ" Johnson, who kept it all together with a smile, and her helpers, Kathi Wise and Rita Teel; Rochelle "RR" Munson and her sister, Janci Farwell, who coordinated all the "aerobic action"; Dr. John Boyer, who always helps keep me safe and semi-sane; the instructors and aerobic dancers who smiled and glowed for freeze frame after freeze frame; Gary Bernstein, whose creative photos make the aerobic lifestyle come alive; Brian Hamilton, for his sunny disposition and creative talents with makeup and hair; John Boswell, my agent, who found the best publisher for my book; Ann Patty, my editor, who convinced me I had something to share; and her super staff who were so enthusiastic about their involvement in this project; Merium Shimp, who diligently typed and re-typed the manuscript; Cynthia Rosen and Marilyn Wabby, who coordinated our "Aerobic Wear" wardrobe and FitnessStuff needs; Herbie Goldstrich and Tom Lichtenwalter, from Lotto Shoes, who made sure all our feet were aerobically dressed; Deborah Szekely, who, years ago, inspired me to improve my eating habits and who continues to do so; Glenn Swengros, my friend, who encouraged me to develop the Everyday Eights; those who always give me loving support: my mommy, Juanita; my step-daddy, Pat; my daddy, Roy; my sister Gayle; my brother Don and his wife, Marcia; my sister Debra, her husband, Allen, and my niece, Tiffany; my cats Runt, Rowdy and Elliott;

And a *standing* ovation for my thousands of instructors all over the world who have inspired hundreds of thousands of students to embrace a lifestyle that's aerobic!

Contents

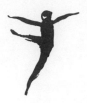

DEFINITIONS

While I still have you sitting down, let's look at the words in the title of this book so you have a better idea of what's ahead.

Jacki Sorensen: That's me, and I'm the originator of Aerobic Dancing, the fitness sport that gives you a head-to-toe workout that's all play.

Aerobic: This word, by itself, simply means "with oxygen," but it comes alive when used as an adjective to describe exercise. Aerobic exercise is exercise that is vigorous enough, lasts long enough and is done regularly enough to keep your heart and your lungs in good shape. More about that later, but I can't wait to tell you that aerobic exercises burn fat faster than any other type of exercise. There's more! The hidden bonus in *aerobic* is the *e*, because it's silent (a-ro-bic) and because it promises excitement, enthusiasm, energy, enjoyment, entertainment, encouragement, and enlightenment!

Lifestyle: This means the style of life you lead, not in terms of whether you drive a luxury car or an old clunk, but how you take care of your body: from eating and exercise to dealing with the everyday challenges of life.

Book: Here it is! Use it, get it sweaty, spill healthy food on it, keep it open by your stereo or refrigerator. But first *read it.*

OVERTURE

This book has been written and produced for:

- Those who received it as a gift from someone who loves them;
- Those who bought it as a gift for themselves because they *care* about themselves;
- Those who are thinking about changing to a healthier, more active lifestyle;
- Those who want to eat without feeling deprived and still lose weight or maintain a healthy, attractive weight;
- Those who exercise regularly but not aerobically;
- Those who exercise aerobically two or three times a week, crave variety, and want to expand to four or five times per week;
- Those who think they're too old to add action to their years;
- Those who are getting older and want to begin or maintain an active lifestyle;
- Those who want to instill healthy lifestyle habits in children and teenagers;
- Those who want to look and feel
   —happier
   —more optimistic
   —more on top of the world!

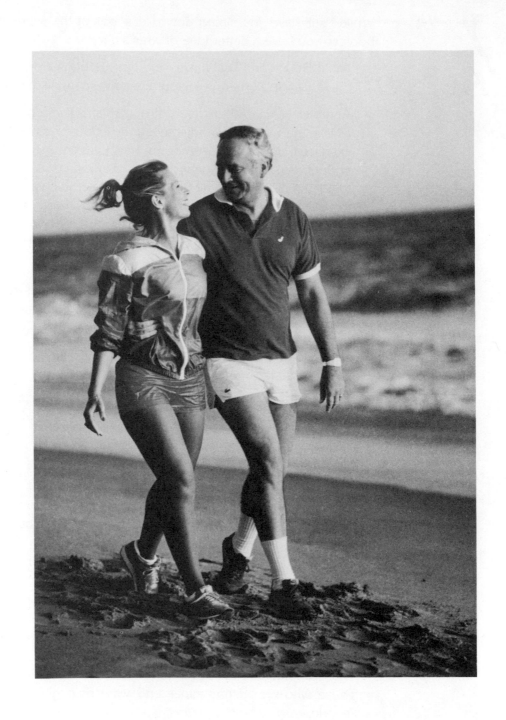

1

The Aerobic Lifestyle

Mark Twain was wrong when he said, "The only way to keep your health is to eat what you don't want, drink what you don't like, and do what you'd rather not." I'm here to replace this negative attitude with a positive approach to acquiring and maintaining a fit, healthy life. My belief is that *movement is life* and you can't be living life to its fullest unless you're as physically fit as you can possibly be. Therefore, my goal Is to motivate you to live a more aerobic lifestyle, no matter how active—or inactive—you may already be.

Here's what being fit means to me: a firm, lean body; a strong heart; a slower heart rate; lower blood pressure; muscle strength; muscle endurance; flexibility; and the most magic ingredient of all: ENERGY. Fitness fever is sweeping the eighties not just because it's good for you, but because it makes you feel so good; so truly alive!

I approach movement as I do life—with enthusiasm, optimism, and style. This is an attitude that can:

- bring joy to every day,
- help you face the daily challenges in life with confidence and a sense of humor,
- inspire you to find aerobic activities that you love,
- motivate you to give up unhealthy habits,
- encourage you to seek improved eating habits,
- help to relieve anxiety and cope with stress,
- and simply make you look better all over.

This is what I mean by an "aerobic lifestyle." I realize your style of living is individual . . . one-of-a-kind, and that my aerobic lifestyle will require adaptation and tailoring to fit your particular needs. That's why I'm not giving you a plan that is programmed out, day by day and week to week. I thrive on spontaneity and being adaptable and I believe that it's this openness to change that's the key to sticking with a lifetime fitness program and a sensible eating plan. What I'm offering are things that I've learned over the years that can be adapted to help you in your own life.

So I have designed this book as your get-it-all-together health and fitness *guide,* built around aerobic exercises such as jogging, cycling, swimming, brisk walking, and Aerobic Dancing—the program I created in 1969. Aerobic exercise involves the whole body, just as the aerobic lifestyle involves your whole style of living. When you put your heart in your exercise, you're rewarded physically, mentally, and emotionally. Aerobic exercise strengthens your heart and lungs while whittling down your fat layer. Brisk participation gives you youthful energy to really *live* instead of just exist. You'll get that glorious feeling of having more energy because exercising aerobically fires you up by requiring you to *use* energy. This may sound paradoxical but it's true, and here's why.

A cardiovascular system that has been conditioned by aerobic exercise becomes more efficient and therefore can work harder for you while expending less energy. This means that you will have energy left over to do other things. Looking at this from another perspective, when you're not active and are under business or personal stress (even the positive stress of happy excitement), adrenaline tends to accumulate in the heart and brain. So, if you feel dragged out after a hard day without exercise, it may be that your system is flooded with adrenaline. An aerobic workout will counteract this excess buildup and leave you feeling refreshed, replenished, and on top of things.

There's a natural high, a feeling of vigor and excitement that exercise provides. With energy reserves you'll be less likely to be in low spirits because you will have more enthusiasm and an ability to do more each day. This may be hard to believe if you're currently living a sedentary life, but you'll believe it when you experience it!

I've motivated millions of Americans to get up and move. Many have written to me that they have regained fitness lost in those transition years from high school through the early years of marriage, getting a career under way, starting a family—or all three. A letter I received from a young housewife in Florida typifies the woman who once thought that a youthful, trim body is lost forever after having a baby. She wrote, ". . . I am now feeling like I used to before I had my first child. Just when I had finally accepted that my body and state of mind would never be the same, I discovered an Aerobic Dancing class and it has returned my life to me."

Another reason for you to embrace the aerobic lifestyle is its carry-over value. Many of my students find that keeping active and fit is a wonderful way to build self-confidence and gain a greater sense of discipline. This in turn gives them impetus and determination to change unhealthy habits. One person told me, "If it hadn't been for your program and the way I was shaping up and feeling so much better about myself, I wouldn't have even considered trying the challenge of giving up smoking."

A regular aerobic program can also open your eyes to what you've been feeding your body, and you'll be motivated to eat more nutritiously as well as more selectively. As one of my students said, "Here I was, going to class every week, and all of a sudden I started asking myself, 'Why am I still eating all this crummy food? I should be trying to feed my body better—I'm an athlete now!' "

Here's the typical evolution I see in so many people when they first begin a regular aerobic program. Initially, they are happily surprised to see inches leave their body. Next, they're excited about new-found energy reserves. And then they're inspired to add a third and fourth day of aerobic activity, even something as simple as walking. After attaining aerobic benefits, they can't wait to expand their fitness horizons. For example, some of our instructors have even tackled the triathlon, where in one continuous race you swim 700 yards, cycle 20 miles, and run 10 miles.

I have six important food and fitness goals in this book that define my concept of the aerobic lifestyle.

FIRST, I want to motivate you to learn a basic set of exercises that can easily be worked into your daily life. Chapter Two will introduce you to my new, original, 15-minute exercise program—the Everyday Eights—that will stretch, tone, and firm your body while giving you aerobic benefits.

SECOND, I want to encourage you to expand your exercise habits to include four aerobic exercise sessions each week. Or, if you're already doing this, why not sample other aerobic activities that will help keep you motivated for life? This variety and flexibility will keep you from becoming a fitness dropout.

THIRD, my students will tell you that it's the fun and excitement of Aerobic Dancing that makes them participate enthusiastically. So, in Chapter Four, you'll learn new Aerobic Dancing *patterns* using some of the favorite, figure-firming steps from my group program. I'll also teach you a new Aerobic *Dance* that will get you hooked on play and style as you get your "chance to dance."

FOURTH, I want to get everybody off "diets" and into improved, realistic eating plans that can take pounds off and keep weight under control. You'll learn ways to gradually acquire healthier eating patterns each year, but eating will still remain enjoyable, non-boring, non-restrictive, and offer the variety which is the essence of a full life. I believe in eating semi-sensibly. That means I'm not an extremist who's out to eliminate all junk food and high-calorie foods from your eating plan. I'm giving you a gentle, reasonable approach . . . and it works! It works because I'm going to allow you to live it up, *provided* you balance your energy output with your eating input. So stick with me until Chapter Six, where I'll give you a wide variety of tips on eating for a trim life.

FIFTH, you'll get straight answers on how to participate actively in a safe and sane way. Dr. John Boyer, my medical consultant, will help me present essential information on stretching, warming up, cooling down, monitoring your heart rates, how to evaluate exercise programs, and which exercise movements to avoid because they are potentially dangerous.

SIXTH, I'll give you some of my philosophy, insights and perspectives that can help you cope with a multifaceted life. I'll talk about ways to balance your many roles and get more done while feeling better about it. We need to learn to accept life with a greater sense of humor and a determination to take time out to smell the flowers, look up to the stars, and reach out to one another. Or, as the lyrics tell us:

> Oh, it's time to start livin'
> Time to take time from the world
>   we're given.
> Time to take time, for Spring
>   will turn to Fall
> In just no time at all.

Many of you have already become a part of the Fitness Generation—and look how far we've come in the last ten or twelve years. For example, when I started Aerobic Dancing as a group program early in 1971, I taught six students in a church basement. Today I have hundreds of thousands of students and I employ over 4,000 instructors. Later in 1971 I ran my first marathon and there were three women in the race. Can you *believe* it— today, when so many thousands of women are running in marathons everywhere? Look how far the fitness revolution has brought us, and yet millions and millions of Americans remain inactive and sedentary. There's still a lot of work to be done. Almost everybody's *interested* in fitness today, but I want to transform that interest into *action*.

If your lifestyle isn't as active—aerobically—as you'd like it to be, don't feel guilty, and don't worry about changing your life overnight. Instead, if you're not happy with the way you look or the way you feel, today is the time to start becoming more active . . . one step at a time. Gradually, progressively, and gently incorporate more exercise and healthier eating habits into your life. Make a few small adjustments and have the patience to realize that a little each day counts, and the little changes you make will add up to something beautiful—a new YOU!

When you make the decision to give up your sedentary ways, you may feel overwhelmed by what seems to lie ahead. Undesirable habits are so ingrained that you can't expect to change your life all at once. So don't despair! Take that first step, and then the second, because that leads to the third and fourth steps, and you're on your way.

> There are mountains in our way
> But we climb a step every day

With all the positive possibilities offered by aerobic activities, why is it such a continual challenge to motivate people to participate and to stick with a program once they begin?

One reason, I know, is the attitude that exercise is an obligation; one more responsibility in an already busy life. Then there's the inconvenience of physical activity on a regular basis, and overcoming sedentary habits that have kept so many people on the sidelines for years, perhaps since childhood. Still another obstacle is the discouragement that comes from doing too much, too soon, too fast. But the excuse I hear the most is: "I don't have enough time to exercise." That argument is lost on me, because I think we all can find the time for something we really *want* to do.

That's why it's so important to think of fitness opportunities as recreation and play, and to find an aerobic approach that's fun for you—a recess from the pressures of life. When exercise in whatever form becomes personally expressive to you, personally satisfying, and a joyful release, you will become addicted to it and you will not want to live without it. Then I'll say, "Welcome to the aerobic lifestyle!"

2

The Everyday Eights

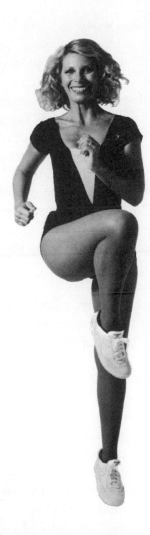

Not since Walter Camp popularized his Daily Dozen in the 1920's has there been a compact, basic fitness program that most people can work into their lifestyle. The Everyday Eights is a brand new, 15-minute exercise program that I've created to give your body a vigorous head-to-toe workout. It's a program for the 1980s that will increase your overall flexibility, improve your muscle tone, exercise you aerobically, and burn fat off your body.

This program was actually motivated by a fractured toe, which occurred shortly before I started a 29-city tour in 1981 to celebrate the tenth anniversary of Aerobic Dancing. Normally, I love to run every day when I'm traveling, for if I feel I'm not getting enough exercise, I tend to get emotionally down instead of being high on life. Since my broken toe would allow me only to walk and do short demonstration dancing on the tour, I knew I needed something to get myself going every morning and to keep my spirits up. So I designed my own daily exercise routine.

Every morning I would get out of bed, tune in the news on television, and then go through a series of flex-and-stretch combos, sit-ups, and movements for all parts of the body. Of course, I also made sure it was aerobic. Then I'd jump in the shower feeling great because I had already done one positive thing for myself. I got another boost knowing it would be easy to fit in one hour of walking later that day, even if I did it in 15-minute segments here and there. Better than sitting in reception rooms waiting to be interviewed!

Surprisingly, a number of the students I met as I traveled across the country wanted a basic exercise workout that they could do at home—a 15 to 20 minute program to use between their Aerobic Dancing classes, or on days when they couldn't get to class. I also met a lot of non-exercisers who just wanted to "get back to basics" when it came to exercise and losing weight. They didn't want to play a sport, but they wanted something effective and enjoyable that they could do every day.

Anxious to fill this need, I went to work on what evolved into the Everyday Eights. I drew on my years of experience as an exercise professional and consulted with my medical advisors in order to develop a basic workout that was safe and motivating.

In 15 minutes you'll cover the main body zones and get your cardiovascular system revved up. In fact, you will have walked or jogged the equivalent of one lap around a 440-yard track: a quarter of a mile!

To make it easier for you to remember the sequence of movements, I've divided this workout into three 5-minute segments.

First, there's the "Head-to-Toe Warm-up," a series of 16 simple moves which warm you up safely and increase and maintain basic flexibility.

Second, you do "Eight for the Floor," a segment which includes stretches to further improve your flexibility and sit-ups to tone and strengthen your abdominal muscles.

Third, you finish with the "Top-to-Bottom Standing Workout," which is a series of movements that strengthen and trim your arms, chest, waist, seat, hips, thighs, and legs. This section is aerobic and it's also individualized, because you can either "walk" this segment or "jog" it.

If you choose the brisk-walk approach in the final segment, all movements are done without jogging, bouncing, or jumping. If you choose the jogging approach, you jog instead of walk and you add "one-steps," bouncing, and jumping to the muscle-toning movements. Both approaches will give you aerobic benefits . . . it's your choice whether you want to be an aerobic walker or an aerobic jogger. What helps make this segment unique and enjoyable is that your walking or jogging is interspersed with figure-toning movements. This adds variety and prevents boredom.

Here's why I'm confident you'll enjoy incorporating the Everyday Eights into your lifestyle:

1. You'll find the movements are easy to memorize because there's a logical pattern to what you are doing.

2. The movements are designed to work your body quickly, safely, and efficiently.

3. You only have to think in eights when it comes to repetitions of a particular movement.

4. Two-thirds of this workout (10 minutes) is done on your feet—which makes exercising more fun. And research shows that this burns slightly more calories than exercising on the floor. So, stand up and move!

5. The Everyday Eights will help you look better by keeping basic muscle groups in shape. Therefore you're going to feel better. And when you feel better and look better, you're going to get more out of life!

6. Even if you're already active, if you aren't doing any special exercises that concentrate on your stomach or upper body, you *need* the

Everyday Eights. Walking and running won't tighten up your stomach muscles, but sit-ups will. And to keep your upper body in shape, I've included a section of arm, chest, and waist exercises.

7. This is an activity that you can do anywhere, in a limited amount of space, and no equipment is needed except shoes. This will pay off on those days when you can't get out of the house to exercise or when you're stuck in a hotel on a business trip. (Even if you're not dressed for exercise, you can do the two standing segments without changing anything but your shoes. Then save the "Eight for the Floor" until later.)

8. This is a family, coed, anybody-can-do-it program. Make it social as well as physical.

9. Take advantage of the Everyday Eights to help maintain your basic flexibility and strength if you have an injury or if you're forced to temporarily forgo your regular exercise program or sporting activities. When you return to your favorite activity, you'll be better prepared to participate—in moderation at first, of course.

10. The Everyday Eights don't *need* music. Neil does them while watching the news in the morning or reruns of M*A*S*H in the evening. However, if you're a music lover, by all means put your favorite songs on the stereo for background music. Just remember to do the Everyday Eights at a speed that's controlled and comfortable for you.

HOW TO USE THE EVERYDAY EIGHTS

I think It's important to have an exercise routine that you can rely upon year after year, no matter what your latest aerobic activity might be, from summer swimming to winter skiing.

The best way to incorporate the Everyday Eights into your current lifestyle would be to do them five days a week, Monday through Friday. This keeps it simple—a workout for your work-week. Once you are thoroughly warmed up, you can expand the aerobic *benefits* into a complete aerobic *workout* by going out for a 30-minute walk or 15 to 20 minutes of jogging. Either is approximately *eight* laps around a track.

You should adjust your use of the Everyday Eights to suit your needs. For example, I'm suggesting that my Aerobic Dancing students who dance on Tuesday and Thursday ought to do the Everyday Eights on Monday, Wednesday and Friday for a body-shaping bonus.

If you're involved in other aerobic programs or activities that fail to tone and trim *all* areas, add regular use of my Everyday Eights to hit those spots that are missed.

And, if you've been living a "healthy" but inactive life, but have decided to start doing something physical that's good for your body, then the Everyday Eights is your answer. You can start out by simply doing this program twice a week, and gradually progress from there. If you never have time to work in anything else physical, you've at least done this one positive thing for your body—and your mind. Give away seven friendly smiles during the day and you can say that you've done *eight* positive things!

So come on! Everyone up for the Everyday Eights! Even if some of you are still saying *No,* that's fine because that's just how the Head-to-Toe Warm-up begins. You say "No" eight times, "Maybe" eight times, and finally "Yes" eight times—and you're on your way!

HEART-RATE MONITORING—YOUR BUILT-IN COACH

When you become an active aerobic lifestyler, heart-rate monitoring should become something you do almost intuitively as part of your workout. Your heart rate is actually a motivating friend when you learn to monitor it properly, for this allows you to objectively detect beneficial changes which you can't otherwise see.

Here are the important terms involved in heart-rate monitoring.

RESTING HEART RATE (RHR): This is taken when you're sitting quietly, and it gives an indication about your level of physical fitness. A person in good aerobic condition usually has a lower resting heart rate compared to that of a person in poor aerobic condition. The average RHR for women is 78–84, and for men, 72–78. A fit heart does not have to beat so often because it can pump more blood with each contraction. This enables it to conserve energy as it does its daily work, and thereby gives you energy reserves.

WORKING HEART RATE (WHR): This is taken during aerobic activity and indicates the level at which your cardiovascular system is performing. This is an excellent indicator of the intensity and effectiveness of your workout. As exercise becomes more vigorous and your muscles require more oxygen, your breathing and heart rate increase. This, in turn, develops aerobic fitness. The WHR should be taken periodically as you exercise.

RECOVERY HEART RATE: This is the measurement taken five minutes after you've stopped exercising. If the count is greater than 120 beats per minute (BPM), you know you've overextended yourself and you need to cut back the intensity of your next workout. After several weeks of aerobic exercise you should find your heart rate returning more quickly to a normal level.

Knowing these basics, here's why heart-rate monitoring is so important.

First, there's the *safety* factor. The heart rate is a gauge by which to assess the intensity of your workout, to make sure you're not overexerting or over-extending yourself. If you take your WHR and you discover that you're above your range, you're exercising too hard and you should slow down.

Second, heart-rate monitoring measures the *effectiveness* of your workout and helps you pace yourself properly. If you are not exercising hard enough (i.e., when your WHR is not within your indicated range in the chart on page 22), then this serves as a built-in coach who's going to inspire you to move out a little more vigorously to get more aerobic benefit from your workout.

If your aerobic activity session is to count as an aerobic *workout* (one of the two-to-four aerobic workouts you should have each week to maintain aerobic fitness), you must stay in your working heart rate range for at least 20 to 30 minutes continuously. So if you're currently in an "aerobics" program, or any exercise program, you can test for yourself to see if you're getting a complete aerobic workout, and not simply some aerobic benefits. If your group leader is not asking students to take their heart rates—or is asking, but not checking the results—then you cannot be assured that this is a true aerobic workout.

In aerobic activities, an important goal is to help the heart become a stronger pump that beats less often but pumps more blood. We accomplish this in Aerobic Dancing by raising the heart rate during class to a safe working range and *maintaining* it for at least 20 to 30 minutes, causing a "training effect" to occur.

Third, taking heart rates gives you an incentive in several important ways. For example, by monitoring your working heart rate from week to week as you participate in an aerobic activity, you'll discover that you will be able to exercise at a higher level of intensity, but at the same or lower WHR. This is the way the heart tells you it is becoming stronger and more efficient.

Another dramatic illustration of what's going on inside your body is offered by the recovery heart rate. When you regularly participate in an aerobic

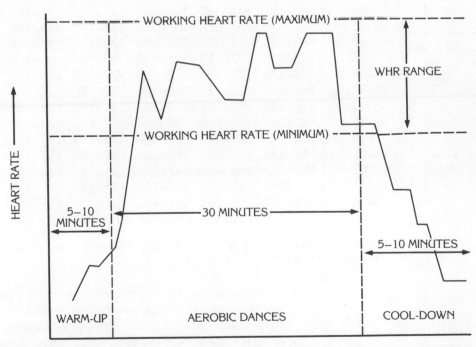

The chart above illustrates the heart rate changes that occur during an Aerobic Dancing class *and is typical of other aerobic workouts*. Notice that the heart rate gradually increases during the warm-up phase, stays within the working heart rate range during the aerobic phase, and gradually returns to "normal" during the cool-down phase. (Adapted from Aerobic Dancing research by Lenore Zohman, M.D.)

activity, notice that your heart begins to recover much more quickly after exercise than it used to. This rapid recovery should give you a motivating lift as you experience yet another indicator that your cardiovascular system is shaping up.

If you're making the transition from a sedentary life to an aerobic lifestyle, you'll most likely find starting out that your heart is an out-of-shape muscle that can barely recover after an aerobic workout. Later, as a result of aerobic conditioning, that same heart has been shaped up as you've shaped up your outer body. You can detect this change by noting how quickly your heart rate returns to normal after a workout, just as you can tell you've lost inches by the way your regular clothes now fit. Heart rate monitoring is the way you "see" the magical changes taking place in your cardiovascular system!

WORKING HEART RATE RANGES

Beats per Minute (BPM)

Resting Heart Rate*	AGE							
	30 and under	31–40	41–45	46–50	51–55	56–60	61–65	65+
50–51	137–195	131–185	128–180	122–170	119–165	116–160	110–150	107–145
52–53	138–195	132–185	129–180	123–170	120–165	117–160	111–150	108–145
54–56	139–195	133–185	130–180	124–170	121–165	118–160	112–150	109–145
57–58	140–195	134–185	131–180	125–170	122–165	119–160	113–150	110–145
59–61	141–195	135–185	132–180	126–170	123–165	120–160	114–150	111–145
62–63	142–195	136–185	133–180	127–170	124–165	121–160	115–150	112–145
64–66	143–195	137–185	134–180	128–170	125–165	122–160	116–150	113–145
67–68	144–195	138–185	135–180	129–170	126–165	123–160	117–150	114–145
69–71	145–195	139–185	136–180	130–170	127–165	124–160	118–150	115–145
72–73	146–195	140–185	137–180	131–170	128–165	125–160	119–150	116–145
74–76	147–195	141–185	138–180	132–170	129–165	126–160	120–150	117–145
77–78	148–195	142–185	139–180	133–170	130–165	127–160	121–150	118–145
79–81	149–195	143–185	140–180	134–170	131–165	128–160	122–150	119–145
82–83	150–195	144–185	141–180	135–170	132–165	129–160	123–150	120–145
84–86	151–195	145–185	142–180	136–170	133–165	130–160	124–150	121–145
87–88	152–195	146–185	143–180	137–170	134–165	131–160	125–150	122–145
89–91	153–195	147–185	144–180	138–170	135–165	132–160	126–150	123–145

* The ideal time to take your resting heart rate (RHR) is before you get out of bed in the morning. Otherwise, make sure you sit quietly for at least 15 minutes.

This chart is based on the medically-proven Karvonen Formula, which uses your age and resting heart rate as a basis, then indicates what your working heart rate range should be in order for you to actually be receiving aerobic benefit. The lower number of each range is the minimum WHR that you should maintain for an aerobic workout. The higher number is the maximum WHR and is used to caution you against over-exertion. However, for safety, we strongly advise you not to exceed 140 BPM during the first two weeks of your first-ever aerobic program.

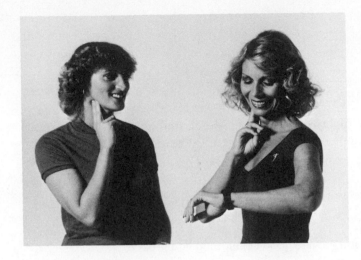

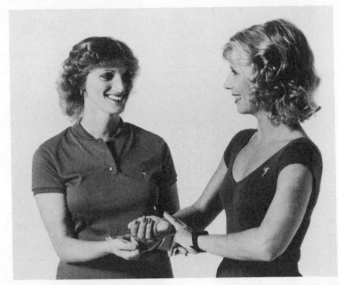

I've always taught people that placing two fingers on the carotid artery in the neck is the easiest way to take their heart rate. Some doctors prefer the pulse to be taken on the thumb side of the inner wrist, and another method is to take your pulse at the temple, but our medical consultant, Dr. John Boyer, says:

"Many people have trouble locating their radial (wrist) pulse, especially quickly, which is important for measuring your working heart rate. Your carotid pulse is stronger and therefore easier to find. Measuring your heart rate in this way does not pose any problem, as long as you do not press on both carotid arteries at the same time, or press too hard. That could produce a heart arhythmia in a tiny percentage of people with coronary disease."

After locating your pulse, keep walking slowly as you count your heart beat for six seconds. This ensures a safe, continuous workout. Add a zero to your count to get your rate per minute, then check that this is within your individual working heart rate range. (See chart, opposite.) It is recommended that you stay below 140 BPM for the first two weeks and then within the lower half of your WHR for the next 10 weeks when beginning an aerobic exercise program.

Working heart rates are taken for six seconds because they drop off fairly rapidly. Resting and recovery heart rates are more constant and should be taken for 15 seconds to ensure an accurate measurement.

SAFETY REMINDERS

Although I've designed the Everyday Eights to provide a safe and efficient workout, here are some hints to maximize the benefits and to help protect yourself from possible injuries:

• Clear a sufficient space to do the workout safely without stubbing your toe or breaking a prized lamp.

• Always wear shoes that are flexible and provide good cushioning and proper support.

• Some people tend to hold their breath while exercising, so don't forget to breathe normally.

• Don't rush the movements. Do each segment at your own pace so you feel in control of each exercise. This helps ensure safe participation while individualizing the workout.

• Remember to practice proper body alignment throughout your workout. Stand tall to show you're a confident, positive person!

• For a thorough, safe workout, it's important to do *all* the movements. If you want to concentrate on a particular area of your body, such as the waistline or your arms, you can gradually and progressively add additional sets of eight repetitions of the appropriate exercise.

• Take your working heart rate immediately at the end of the final segment, before you start your cool-down. You've just finished your aerobic phase and it's important to monitor what your heart is doing.

The Everyday Eights—Segment I

HEAD-TO-TOE WARM-UP

1. Stand with your feet comfortably spaced, arms down at your sides, shoulders back and down. Keep your feet spaced this way unless directions tell you to do otherwise.

2. "Feet together" means just what it says.

3. "Feet in stride position" means feet just a little bit wider than shoulder-width apart.

1. Say "No"

8 times slowly

Body benefits: stretches neck muscles and releases tension

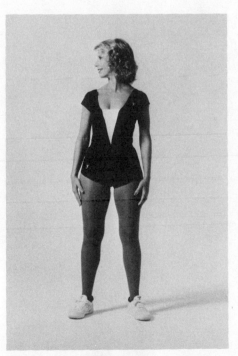

Turn head to right, then

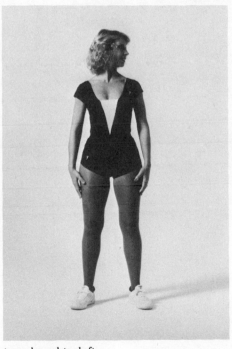

turn head to left.

THIS IS ONE TIME.

2. Say "Maybe"

8 times slowly

Body benefits: stretches neck muscles
and releases neck tension

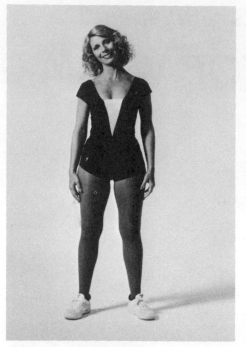 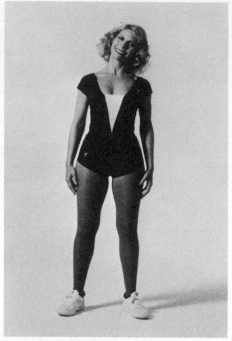

Tilt head to right, then   tilt head to left.

THIS IS ONE TIME.

3. Say "Yes"

8 times slowly

Body benefits: stretches neck muscles
and releases neck tension

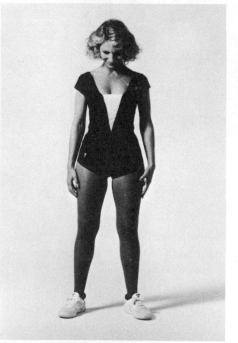 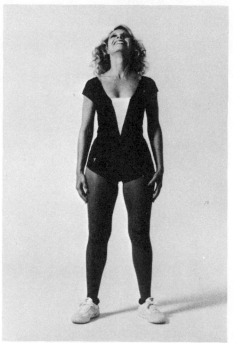

Gently drop chin down, then   gently lift chin up.

THIS IS ONE TIME.

26

4. Shoulder Rolls, Single

8 times

Body benefits: stretches and loosens shoulder muscles and releases shoulder tension

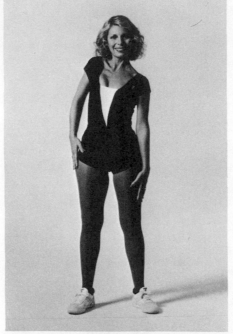 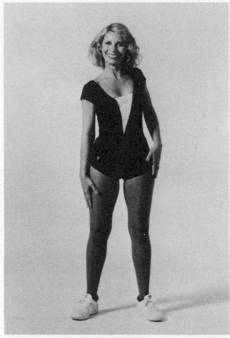

Roll right shoulder up, back, down and around with a continuous motion, then repeat the movement to the left, rolling left shoulder up, back, down and around with a continuous motion.

THIS IS ONE TIME.

5. Shoulder Rolls, Double

8 times

Body benefits: stretches and loosens shoulder muscles and upper back

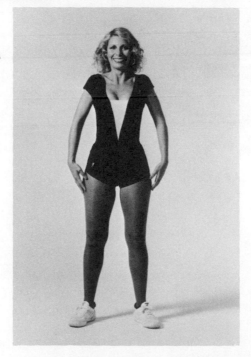

Roll both shoulders up, back, down and around with a continuous motion.

THIS IS ONE TIME.

6. Pull-Back Stretch

8 times

Body benefits: stretches chest, scapula, upper back and upper arms

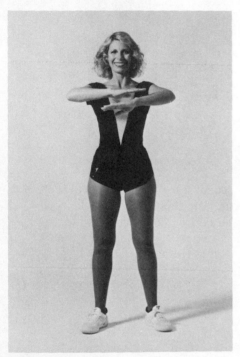 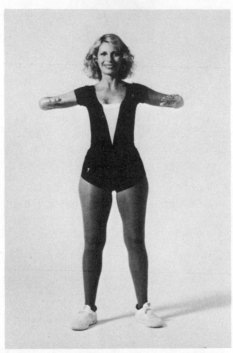 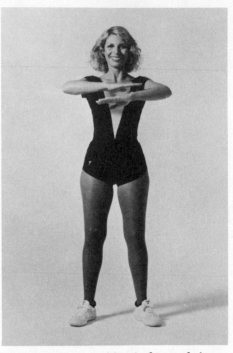

Begin with elbows bent, hands extended approximately 18″ in front of chest.

Gently pull elbows back, keeping back straight, then

return arms to position in front of chest.

THIS IS ONE TIME.

Do the first six Head-to-toe Warm-up movements any time, anywhere, to relieve tension in your neck and shoulders, or just as a quick and refreshing perk-yourself-up break.

7. Side Bends

8 times

Body benefits: stretches waist and sides of body

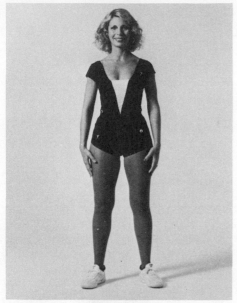 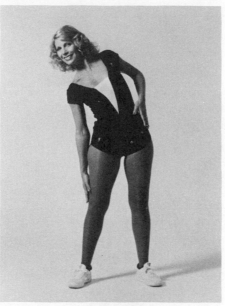 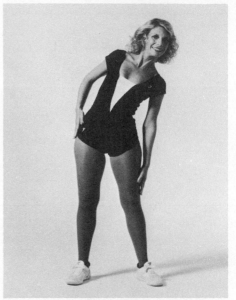

With feet in stride position, arms down at sides,

gently bend to the right. Return, then

gently bend to the left. Return.

THIS IS TWO TIMES.

8. Low Back Twist

8 times

Body benefits: stretches sides of body and lower back

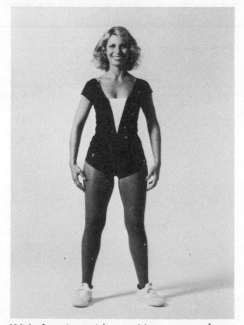 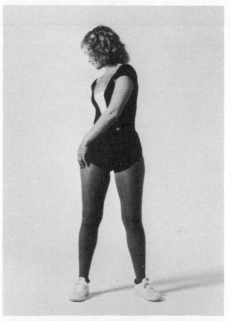 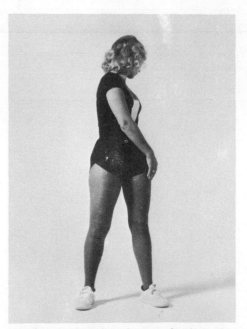

With feet in stride position, arms down at sides,

gently twist head and upper body to the right so you can see your heels, then

gently twist head and upper body to the left, and look at your heels.

HURRAH FOR YOU! YOU'RE HALFWAY THROUGH THE WARM-UPS!

THIS IS TWO TIMES.

9. Knee-Bend Stretch

8 times

Body benefits: stretches upper body and arms while preparing (warming up) your knees and legs for more vigorous exercises to follow

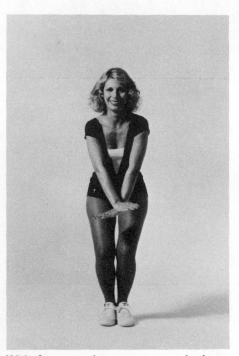 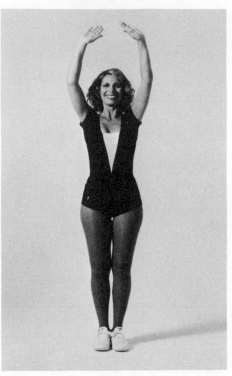 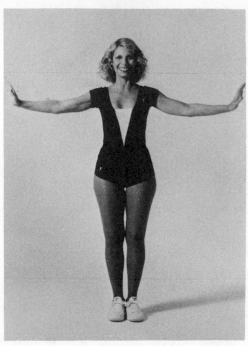

With feet together, arms stretch down and cross as knees bend slightly, then

arms circle across body and stretch up as knees straighten,

and continue circling around to end out at sides.

THIS IS ONE TIME.

10. Sporty Stretch

8 slow counts to each side

Body benefits: stretches inner thigh muscles

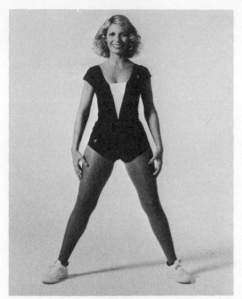 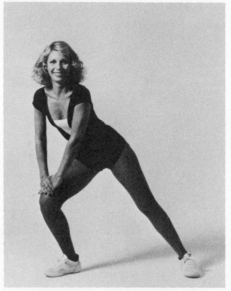 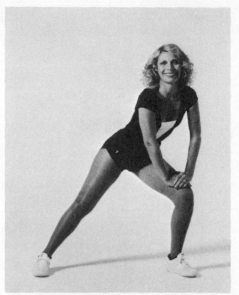

With feet approximately three feet apart, turn the right foot to face right diagonal; the left foot faces forward. Bend right knee and place hands above it with elbows slightly bent. Both feet are flat on the floor and weight is evenly distributed. Hold 8 slow counts.

Reverse, bending left knee with left foot facing left diagonal, right foot facing forward. Hold 8 slow counts.

11. Flamingo Fling

8 slow counts for each leg

Body benefits: stretches quadricep muscles

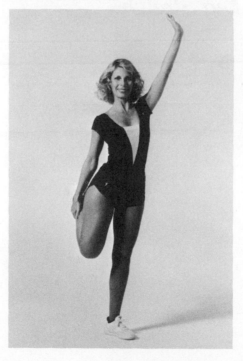 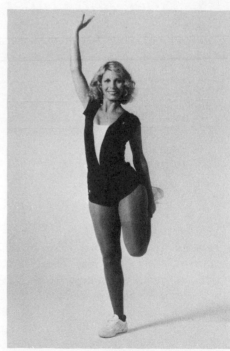

Place left hand on wall or chair, or practice keeping your balance and hold it overhead. Raise right foot behind body and grasp ankle with right hand. Holding on to your ankle, gently bring right knee back in line with left leg and hold this stretch for 8 slow counts.

Reverse stance, using right arm for balance, bending left knee. Hold for 8 slow counts.

12. Hamstring Stretch

2 times

Body benefits: stretches hamstrings and back muscles

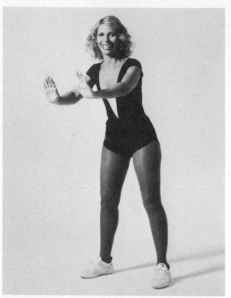

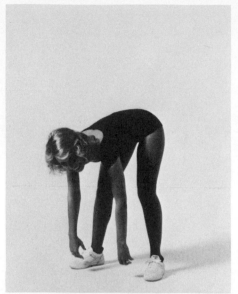

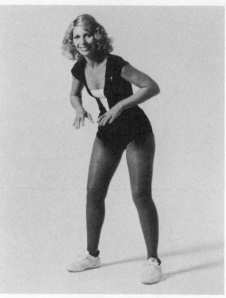

With feet in stride position, arms bent in front of chest, push arms forward, then

gently bend forward at waist with knees relaxed and chin up. Bend as far as is comfortable. Hold for 8 slow counts. (It's not necessary to touch floor or toes.)

Slowly straighten, bending knees slightly to take pressure off the lower back and return to starting position.

THIS IS ONE TIME.

13. Knee and Lower Leg Stretch

4 outward circles and 4 inward circles for each leg

Body benefits: stretches knee, calf, and ankle

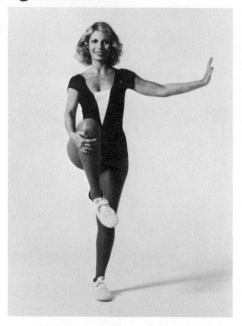

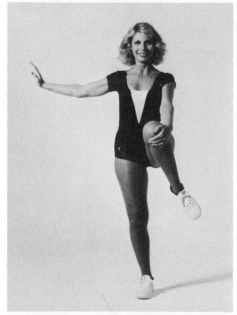

Place left hand on wall or chair, or practice keeping your balance with left arm extended out to the side. Raise right knee and gently grasp below knee with right hand. Rotate lower leg and foot outward to make 4 circles, then inward to make 4 circles.

Reverse stance, using right arm for balance, circling left lower leg and foot. (Now you've done 8 circles with each leg.)

14. Calf Stretch

8 slow counts for each leg

Body benefits: stretches calf and ankle

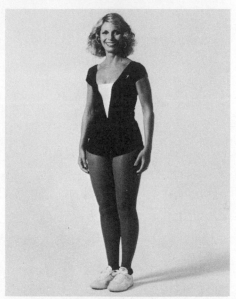

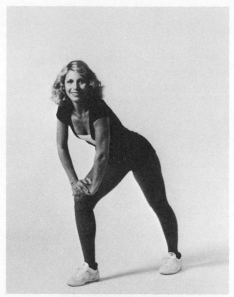

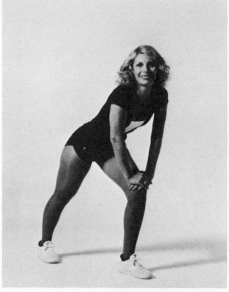

Stand with feet together and keep both feet pointed forward *throughout*.

Take a big step forward with right foot, bending right knee, keeping left leg straight, and placing both hands above right knee with arms straight. Hold 8 slow counts then return to starting position.

Reverse stance, stepping forward with left foot, left knee bent, hands placed above left knee, and right leg straight. Hold 8 slow counts then return to starting position.

15. Foot Stretches

4 outward circles and 4 inward circles for each foot

Body benefits: Stretches the 19 muscles in your feet! (Can you believe you have this many?) The foot contains 26 bones and 33 articulations joined together by over 100 ligaments. Nineteen muscles provide power and control of the foot.

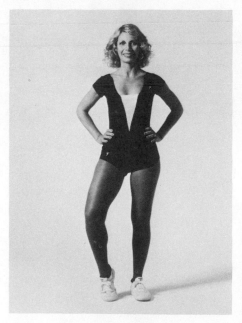

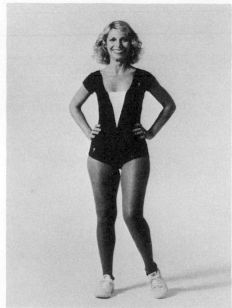

With hands placed on hips and feet slightly apart, shift weight to left leg and rotate right foot outward to make 4 circles, then inward to make 4 circles.

Reverse, circling left foot. (Now you've done 8 circles with each foot.)

16. On Your Toes

(You made it!) —8 times

Body benefits: stretches calf, ankle and foot

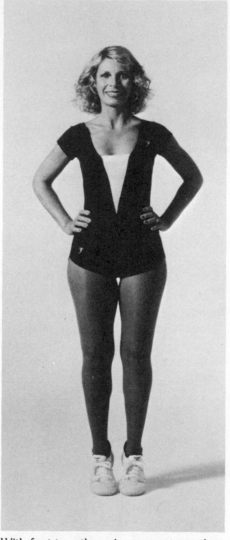 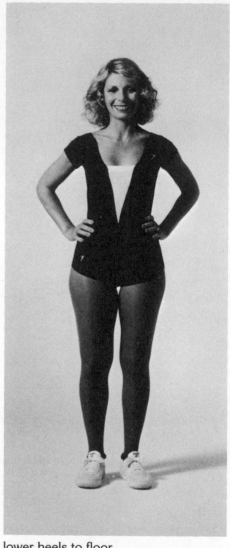

With feet together, rise up on toes, then lower heels to floor.

THIS IS ONE TIME.

The Everyday Eights—Segment II
EIGHT FOR THE FLOOR

If you need a softer surface, use a mat
or towel for your floor workout.

This is one way to get there!

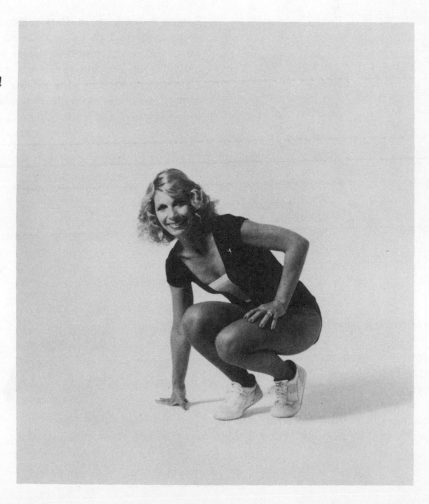

1. Static Stretch

Body benefits: stretches back, hamstrings and inner thighs

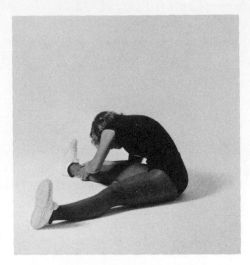

Right Leg Flexibility—*8 slow counts*

Seated in medium stride position, turn upper body to face right foot, bend forward from waist, lowering upper body toward your leg, and grasp lower leg. Be sure to keep legs straight, toes upright. (It's not necessary to touch head to leg.) Hold for 8 slow counts.

Left Leg Flexibility—*8 slow counts*

Seated in medium stride position, turn upper body to face left foot, bend forward from waist, lowering upper body toward your leg, and grasp lower leg. Be sure to keep legs straight, toes upright. (It's not necessary to touch head to leg.) Hold 8 slow counts.

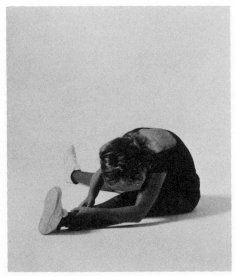

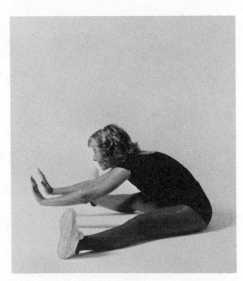

Forward Flexibility—*8 slow counts*

Seated in medium stride position, gently bend forward from the waist, lowering upper body toward the floor as far as you can without strain, arms stretched out in front. Be sure to keep legs straight, toes upright. Hold 8 slow counts.

2. Knee Pull

8 times, alternating right and left, 2 slow counts each

Body benefits: stretches lower back and legs

Lie on back with knees relaxed, arms down at sides.

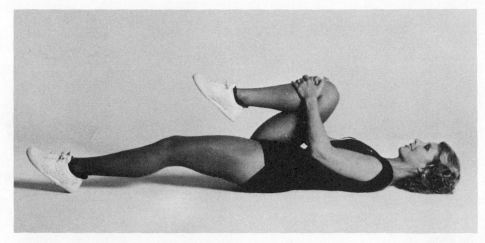

Lift right knee close to chest, grasp lower leg, and gently pull knee toward chest, then

return right leg to starting position as hands gently hit floor next to hips.

THIS IS ONE TIME.

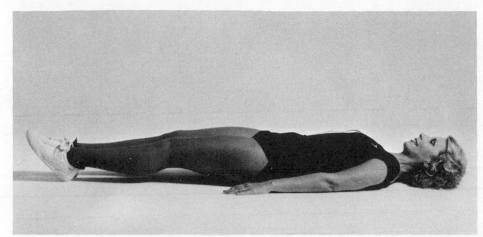

Reverse, using left leg.

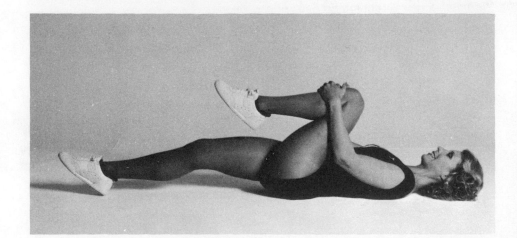

3. Lower Back Flexibility Roll

8 times, slowly

Body benefits: increases flexibility in lower back and strengthens abdominal muscles

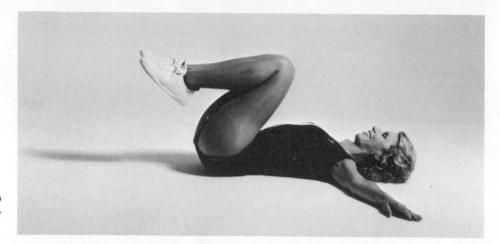

Lie on back with knees bent close to chest, arms extended out at sides for support.

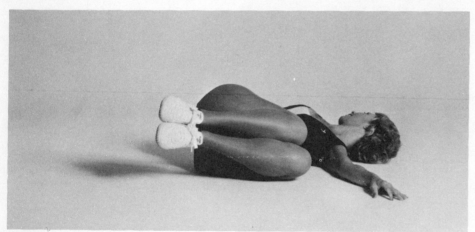

Keeping shoulders on the floor, roll to left hip, knees touching to left side, head looking to right. Return to starting position, then

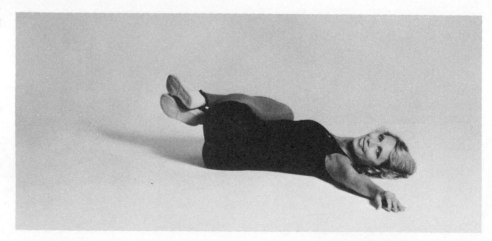

keeping shoulders on the floor, roll to right hip, knees touching to right side head looking to left side. Return to starting position.

THIS IS TWO TIMES.

4. Wringers

8 times

Body benefits: stretches neck, sides of body, lower back, hamstring of lifted leg, and increases hip and lower back flexibility

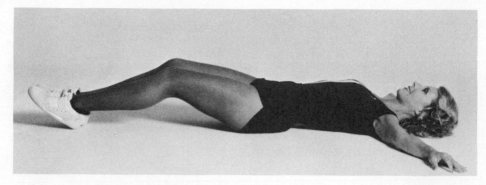

Lie on your back with knees relaxed, arms extended out at sides for support.

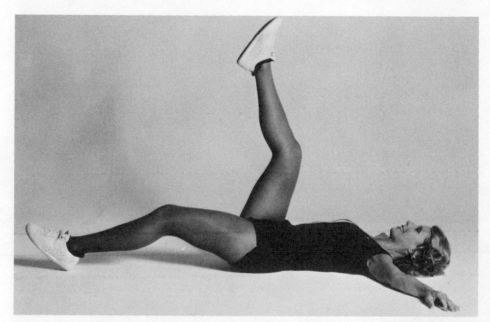

Raise right leg over body, keeping knees relaxed.

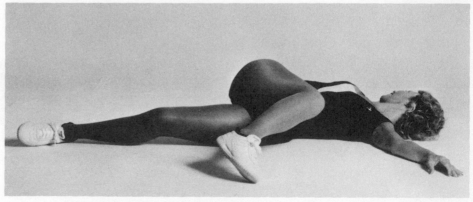

Stretch right leg across body to the left, touching foot to floor. Head looks to right. Then

raise right leg back over body and lower to starting position.

THIS IS ONE TIME.

Reverse, using left leg.

5. Side Leg Raisers

8 times with right leg, then 8 times with left leg

Body benefits: stretches ankle and inner and outer thighs

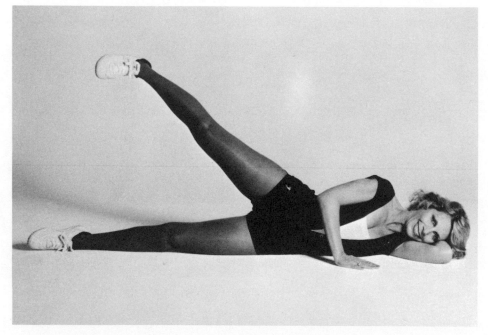

Lie on left side with head resting comfortably on arm in line with spine. Place right hand on floor in front of you for support. Point your right foot toward the floor.

Raise right leg 24 to 36 inches, keeping toes pointed toward floor.

Lower right leg so toes gently touch the arch of the resting foot.

THIS IS ONE TIME.

Roll to right side and repeat with the left leg.

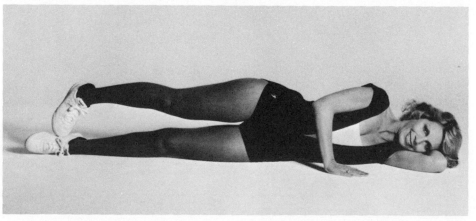

6. The Cat

8 times to the right, then return to starting position and 8 times to the left

Body benefits: strengthens abdominals and back, and increases hip flexibility (you know how flexible cats are!)

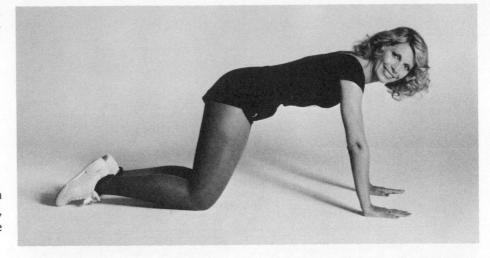

Kneel on your hands and knees with weight evenly distributed, back straight, abdominals pulled in and head in line with spine.

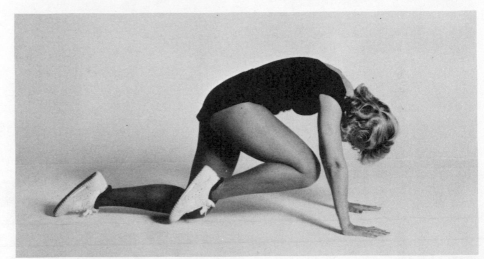

Gently drop head down and round your back ("curl up") as right knee pulls in toward chest.

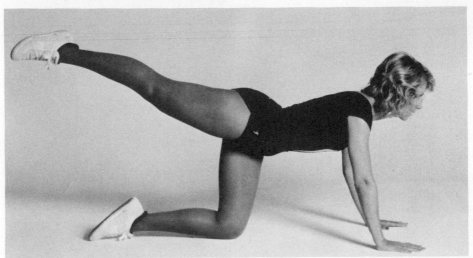

Head lines up with spine as right knee straightens, leg lifts up in back *a bit*, and you stretch out.

THIS IS ONE TIME.

Return to starting position and reverse, using left leg.

7. Low Back Stretch

Do once.

Body benefits: stretches lower back and buttocks

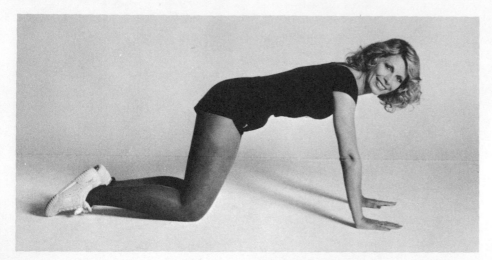

Kneel on hands and knees with weight evenly distributed, back straight, abdominals pulled in, and head in line with spine.

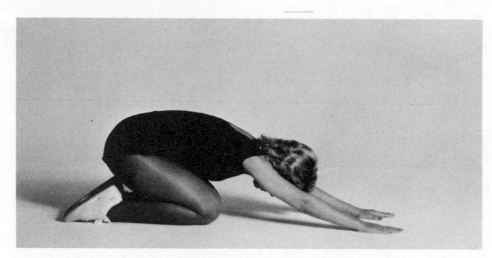

Sit back on your heels, lowering chest toward the floor, keeping hands on the floor out in front of you, and drop head. Hold for 8 slow counts.

8A. Sit-Up Touch

8 times

Body benefits: strengthens and firms the abdominal muscles

In the beginning do as many sit-ups as you can comfortably handle. Then add one sit-up at a time (at your own pace) until you reach your ultimate goal of 32 sit-ups. Train, don't strain, your abdominal muscles.

When doing sit-ups, remember to do them with a slow, smooth and controlled motion.

If you are not able to do a complete sit-up at first, simply curl up as far as you can, hold for two counts, then curl down.

Lie on back with knees bent, feet flat on floor or resting on heels, arms extended on the floor past your head with elbows relaxed.

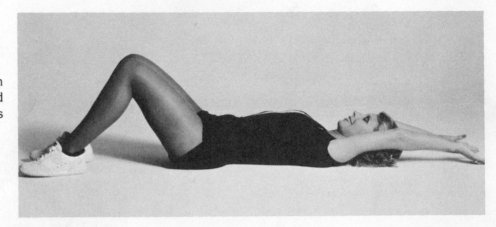

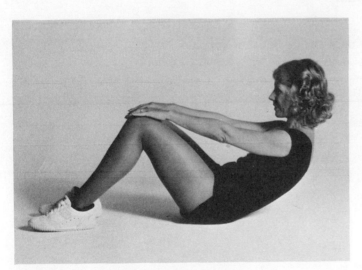

Count one: Tucking head, curl up slowly and touch knees with fingertips.

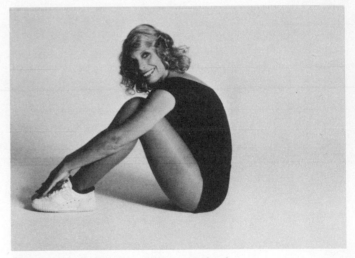

Count two: Continue curling up slowly and touch feet with fingertips as you lean forward.

(continued)

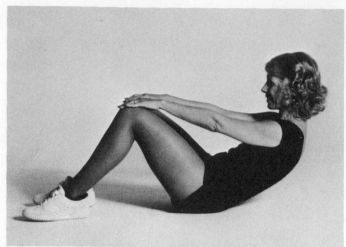

Count three: Touch knees again as you begin curling down slowly.

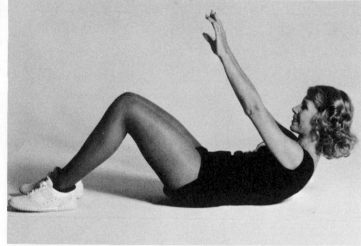

Count four: Continue curling down slowly as you return to starting position.

THESE FOUR SLOW COUNTS EQUAL ONE TIME.

8B. Sit-Up Twist

8 times, alternating right and left

Body benefits: strengthens and firms abdominal muscles, trims the waist and increases lower back flexibility

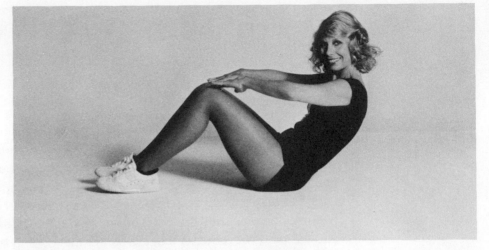

Count one: From same starting position, tucking head, curl up slowly and touch knees with fingertips.

Count two: Keeping back straight, gently twist upper body to right side with elbows bent, hands extended approximately 18″ in front of chest.

Count three: Touch knees again as you begin curling down slowly.

Count four: Continue curling down slowly as you return to starting position.

THESE FOUR SLOW COUNTS EQUAL ONE TIME.

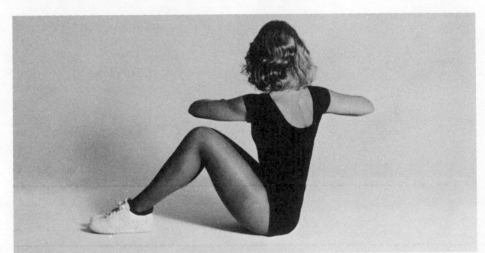

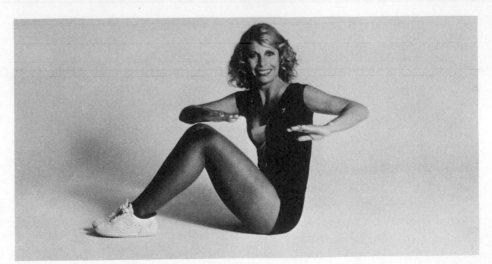

Reverse, sitting up and gently twisting upper body to left side.

REPEAT SIT-UP TOUCH—8 TIMES SLOWLY

REPEAT SIT-UP TWIST—8 TIMES SLOWLY, ALTERNATING RIGHT AND LEFT

TOP-TO-BOTTOM WORKOUT

(Brisk Walking Level)

The first two segments of the Everyday Eights have been the same for everyone. Now I'm giving you a choice of two approaches to this final segment: a brisk walking level or a jogging level. As a safety factor the first time, I want you to go through this at the walking level, even if you intend to take the jogging approach. It's not only safer but also easier to become familiar with the basic exercises *before* adding the bouncing and jumping movements that are part of the jogging level.

1. Always stand with your feet comfortably spaced, unless the directions tell you to do otherwise. "Feet together" means just what it says; "feet in stride position" means your feet should be a little bit *wider* than shoulder-width apart.

2. Always begin the exercises with your abdominals pulled in and up, shoulders back and down, and seat tucked under.

3. I want you to cover ground when you walk, rather than simply walking in place. It's safer and more natural to "move out" in circles or, ideally, from room to room.

1A. Arm Circles, Pushed Out

8 times forward, 8 times backward

Body benefits: strengthens and firms muscles in upper and lower arms

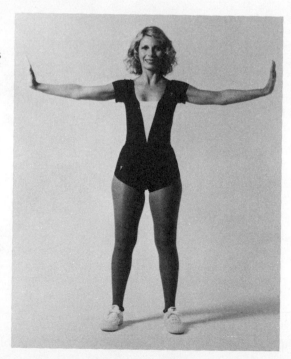

Extend arms out at sides, shoulder height, with wrists flexed back, palms open and facing out. Smoothly rotate arms in medium-sized circles. The circling involves the whole arm and is done with a continuous motion.

1B. Arm Circles, Closed Down

8 times forward, 8 times backward

Body benefits: strengthens and firms muscles in upper and lower arms

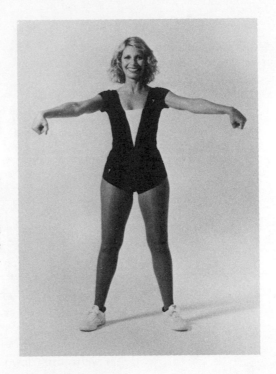

Extend arms out at sides, shoulder height, with hands in loose fists, dropped down from the wrists. Smoothly rotate arms in medium-sized circles. The circling involves the whole arm and is done with a continuous motion.

2. Rope-Climbing

8 times

Body benefits: strengthens waist, sides of body and arms

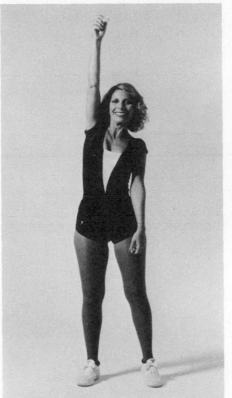 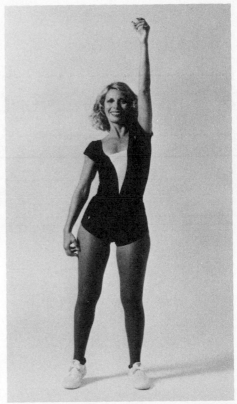

Reach up overhead with your right arm then pull your right arm down with a bent elbow.

Reach up overhead with your left arm then pull your left arm down with a bent elbow. Use your inner body strength to feel as if you are pulling yourself up a rope.

THIS IS TWO TIMES.

3. *Backstroke*

8 times

Body benefits: stretches sides of body, waist, arms and increases shoulder and lower back flexibility

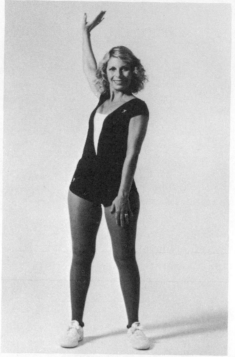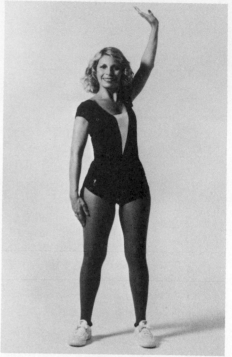

Begin with arms down, hands resting on front of thighs. Reach right arm forward, up, around and down behind you with a smooth continuous motion and end with hand resting on front of right thigh.

Reach left arm forward, up, around and down behind you with a smooth continuous motion and end with hand resting on front of left thigh. You should feel as if you are doing the backstroke.

THIS IS TWO TIMES.

4. *Snap-Down, Front*

8 times

Body benefits: strengthens and firms arms and pectoral muscles

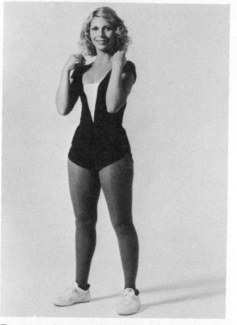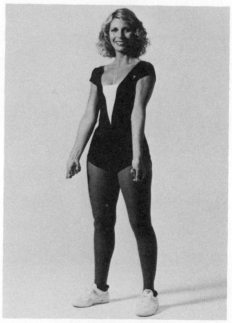

Begin with arms bent and held at your waist ("jogging arms"). Hands move up in front of shoulders in loose fists as your elbows lift forward, then

forearms extend forward and down as you straighten your elbows, snap your fingers, and end with hands in front of thighs.

THIS IS ONE TIME.

48

5. Snap-Behind

8 times

Body benefits: strengthens and firms arms and pectoral muscles

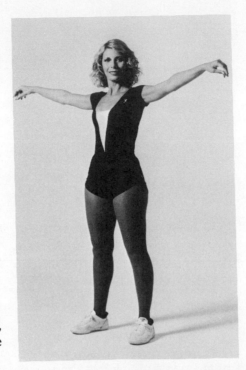

Begin with arms held out at sides, shoulder height, with hands in loose fists, shoulders back and down.

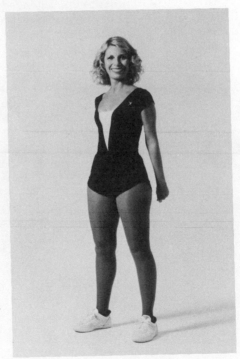

Swing arms down at sides to end behind buttocks with a snap of your fingers. Swing arms back to end out at shoulder level.

THIS IS ONE TIME.

6. *Criss-Cross*

4 counts low to high
4 counts high to low
4 counts low to high
4 counts high to low

Body benefits: stretches and firms arms and pectoral muscles

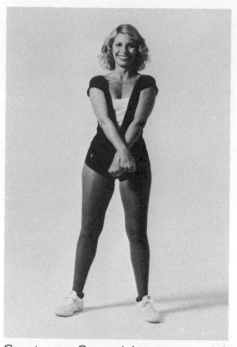

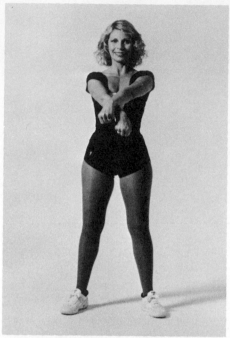

Begin with arms extended down from the shoulders in a wide-open "V" in front of body, hands in loose fists.

Count one: Cross right arm over left arm at lower arms. Uncross and open arms to end extended in a wide "V" in front of body at waist level.

Count two: Cross left arm over right arm, crossing lower arms at chest level. Uncross and open arms to end extended in a wide "V" in front of body at chest level.

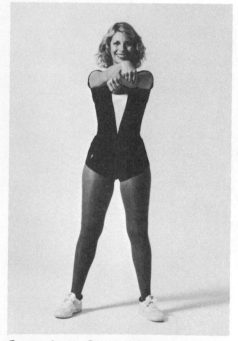

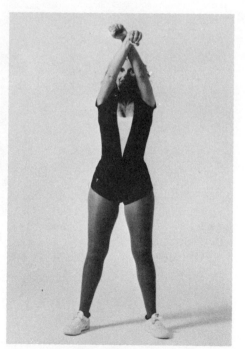

Count three: Cross right arm over left arm, crossing lower arms at shoulder level. Uncross and open arms to end extended in a wide "V" in front of body at shoulder level.

Count four: Cross left arm over right arm, crossing lower arms above the head. Uncross and open arms to end extended in a "V" in front of body at head level.

Continue, beginning the Criss-Cross at head level and lowering arms to end down in front of abdomen.

7. Side Bends

Do a total of 32, following this sequence:
8 times to the right
8 times to the left
4 times to the right
4 times to the left
2 times to the right
2 times to the left
2 times to the right
2 times to the left

Body benefits: stretches your waist and upper body and increases flexibility in the lower back

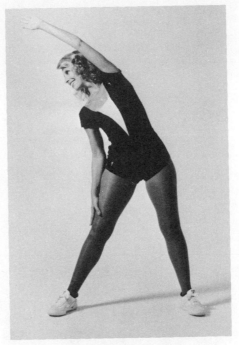

Stand with feet in stride position, left arm overhead and right arm down at side, hand resting loosely on thigh. Bend smoothly to the right keeping right arm on thigh for support. Return to the upright position.

THIS IS ONE TIME TO THE RIGHT.

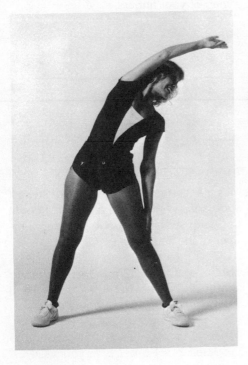

Repeat according to the pattern above, then reverse, bending to the left, and continue following pattern.

8. Twist and Snap

8 times, alternating right and left

Body benefits: stretches and firms upper body and increases flexibility in the lower back

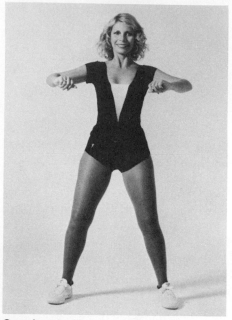

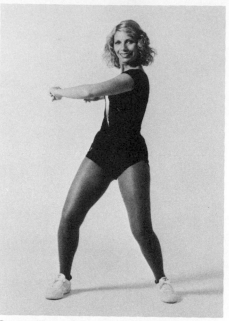

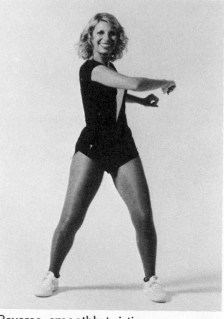

Stand with feet in stride position and knees slightly bent, hands extended approximately 18″ in front of chest with elbows bent.

Smoothly twist arms and upper body and head to the right side with a snap of your fingers.

THIS IS ONE TIME.

Reverse, smoothly twisting arms, upper body, and head to the left side with a snap of your fingers.

9. Stroll Walk

8 sets of 8 steps

Body benefits: aerobic!

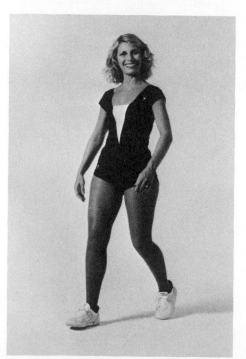

Stand tall with abdominals pulled in and up.

Whenever possible, do not walk in place! Move around as you walk and try to vary your route from day to day. Pick up and carry things that need to be moved from one room to another. This way you'll be a "step ahead" in your housework!

It's a snap to count the 8 sets of steps if you snap your fingers on the first count of each set and say out loud the number of the set.

Snap and say "One," then count to yourself 2-3-4-5-6-7-8, as you take 8 steps;

snap and say "Two," then count to yourself 2-3-4-5-6-7-8, as you walk.

Continue until you complete eight sets.

52

10. Knee-Lift Combo

Do 32 in this sequence:
8 times forward
8 times crossing
8 times forward
8 times open

Body benefits: front of thighs, back of thighs, and seat

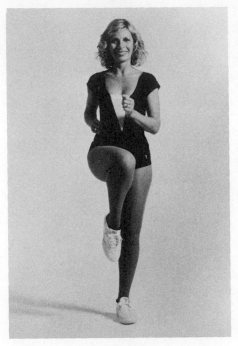 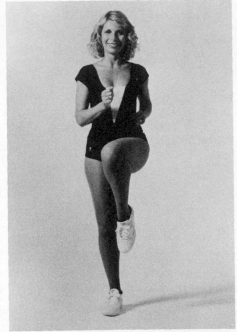

Knee-Lift, Forward—*8 times, alternating right and left.*

Lift your right knee up *in front,* then put your right foot down next to your left foot.

THIS IS ONE TIME.

Lift your left knee up *in front,* then put your left foot down next to your right foot.

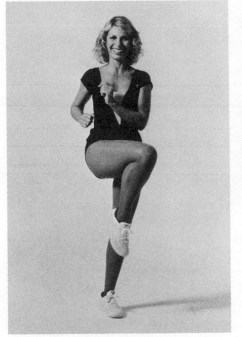 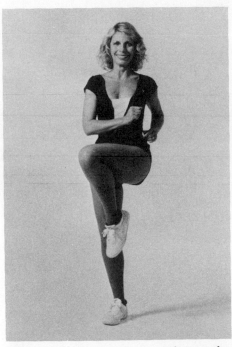

Knee-Lift, Crossing—*8 times, alternating right and left*

Lift your right knee up to *point to the left diagonal,* then put your right foot down next to your left foot.

THIS IS ONE TIME.

Lift your left knee up *to point to the right diagonal,* then put your left foot down next to your right foot.

(continued)

Knee-Lift Combo (continued)

Knee-Lift, Forward—*8 times, alternating right and left.*

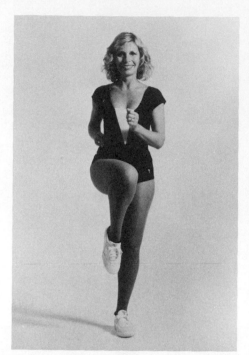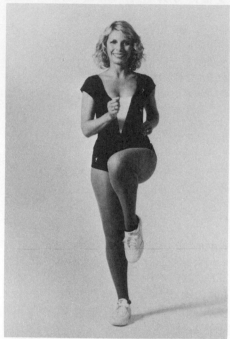

Lift your right knee up *in front,* then put your right foot down next to your left foot.

THIS IS ONE TIME.

Lift your left knee up *in front,* then put your left foot down next to your right foot.

Knee-Lift, Open—*8 times, alternating right and left*

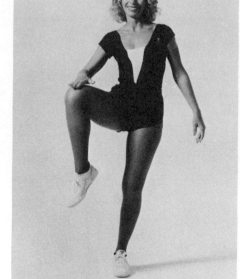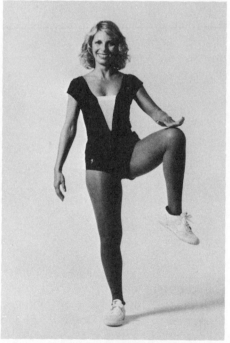

Lift your right knee up to point *to the right diagonal,* hitting the top of your right thigh gently with your right hand. Then put your right foot down next to your left foot.

THIS IS ONE TIME.

Lift your left knee up to point *to the left diagonal,* hitting the top of your left thigh gently with your left hand. Then put your left foot down next to your right foot.

11. Brisk Walk

8 sets of 8 steps

Body benefits: aerobic!

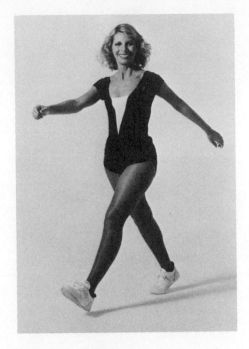

Move out with more vigor—

Step lively—

Walk energetically!

12. Kick Combo

Do 32 kicks in this sequence:
8 forward
8 crossing
8 forward
8 open

Body benefits: legs, front of thighs, back of thighs, inner and outer thighs, and seat

Kick, Forward—*8 times, alternating right and left*

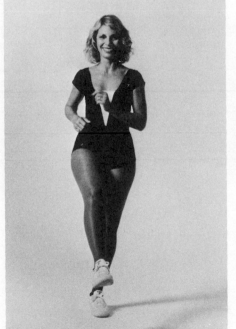

Kick your right foot *forward low* (no higher than waist level), then put your right foot down next to your left foot.

THIS IS ONE TIME.

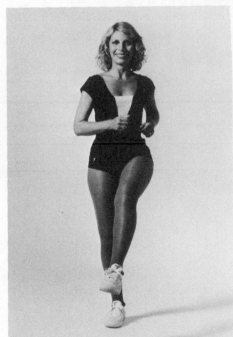

Kick your left foot *forward low* (no higher than waist level), then put your left foot down next to your right foot.

(continued)

Kick Combo (continued)

Kick, Crossing—*8 times, alternating right and left*

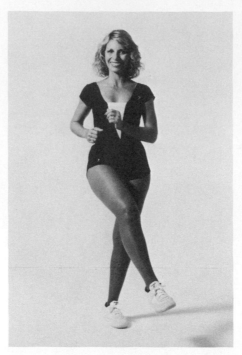 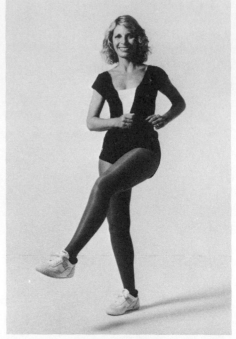

Kick your right foot forward low *to the left diagonal* (no higher than waist level), then put your right foot down next to your left foot.

THIS IS ONE TIME.

Kick your left foot forward low *to the right diagonal* (no higher than waist level), then put your left foot down next to your right foot.

Kick, Forward—*8 times, alternating right and left*

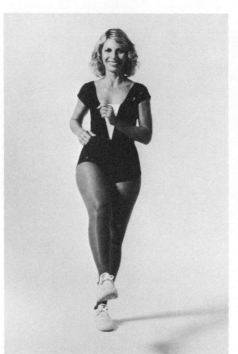 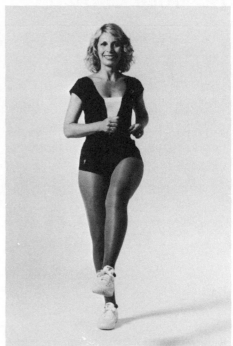

Kick your right foot *forward low* (no higher than waist level), then put your right foot down next to your left foot.

THIS IS ONE TIME.

Kick your left foot *forward low* (no higher than waist level), then put your left foot down next to your right foot.

Kick, Open—*8 times, alternating right and left*

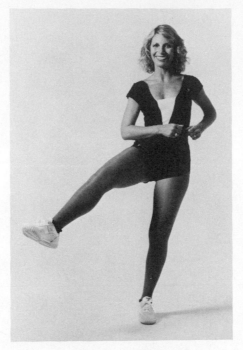 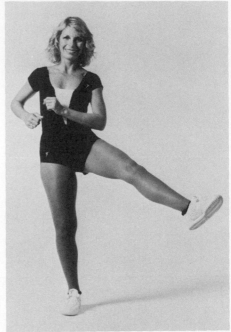

Kick your right foot forward low *to the right diagonal* (no higher than waist level), then put your right foot down next to your left foot.

THIS IS ONE TIME.

Kick your left foot forward low *to the left diagonal* (no higher than waist level), then put your left foot down next to your right foot.

13. Brisk Walk

8 sets of 8 steps

Body benefits: aerobic!

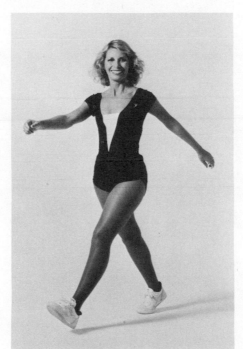

When you've finished this brisk walk you will have walked more than halfway around a quarter-mile track! You're on the home stretch!

14. Side Leg-Lifts

16 times, alternating right and left

Body benefits: inner and outer thighs

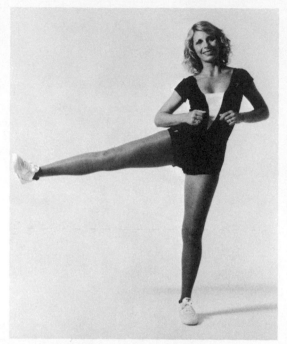

Lift your right leg out to the right side as high as is comfortable, then

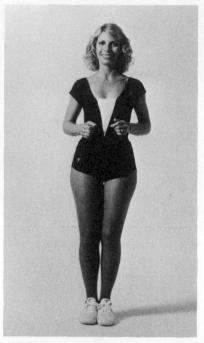

bring your right foot down next to your left foot.

THIS IS ONE TIME.

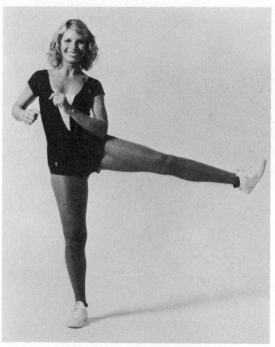

Lift your left leg out to the left side as high as is comfortable, then

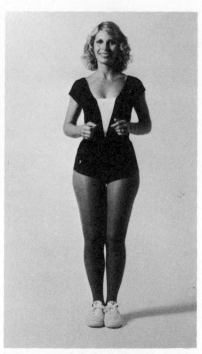

bring your left foot down next to your right foot.

15. Brisk Walk

8 sets of 8 steps

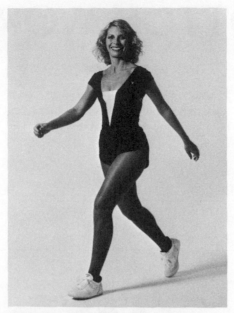

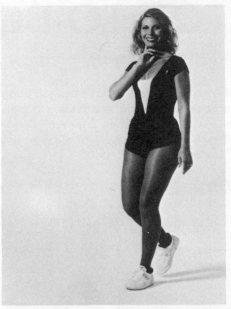

Maintain posture—
Walk with a lilt . . . and a smile—
Lift those knees a bit.

Take your working heart rate.

NOTE: At this point, expand your aerobic benefits into a complete aerobic workout by taking a 30-minute walk. (Approximately 8 laps around a track.)

16. Cool-Down

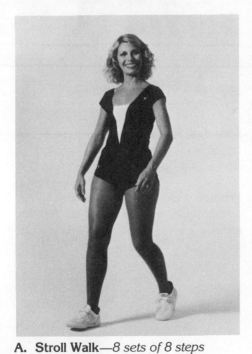

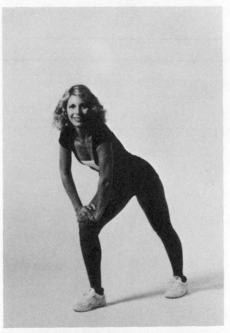

With feet together, keeping both feet pointing forward throughout, take a big step forward with right foot, bending right knee and keeping left leg straight. Place both hands above right knee with arms straight. Hold for 8 slow counts; then return to starting position.

Reverse stance, stepping left foot forward to stretch your right calf. Hold for 8 slow counts.

Take your recovery heart rate.

A. Stroll Walk—*8 sets of 8 steps*

You've just walked ¼ mile!
GOOD FOR YOU!

B. Calf Stretch—*8 slow counts for each leg*

TOP-TO-BOTTOM WORKOUT

(Jogging Level)

1. At this level, you'll be jogging, bouncing, jumping and adding "One-Steps" to movements 1 through 6, so first I'll teach you what a "One-Step" is.

2. Always begin the exercises with your abdominals pulled in and up, shoulders back and down, and seat tucked under.

3. I want you to move out and cover as much distance as you can when you jog. This is safer and more enjoyable than jogging in place.

One-Step

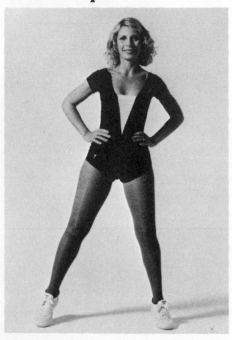

Begin with feet together, hands on hips. Step **right** with right foot, then

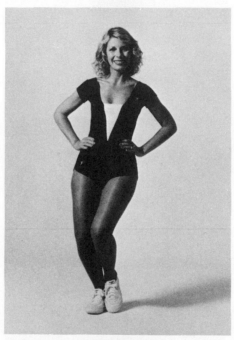

draw **left** foot in to right foot

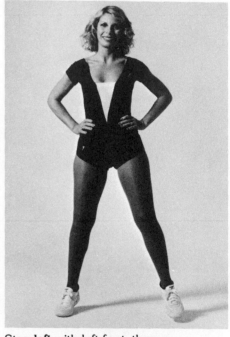

Step **left** with left foot, then

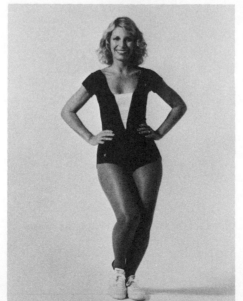

draw **right** foot in to left foot.

THIS IS TWO ONE-STEPS.

Practice these One-Steps until you feel comfortable, and then start adding the arms.

1A. One-Step Arm Circles, Pushed Out

8 times forward; this takes 4 One-Steps
8 times backward; this takes 4 One-Steps

Body benefits: strengthens and firms muscles in upper and lower arms

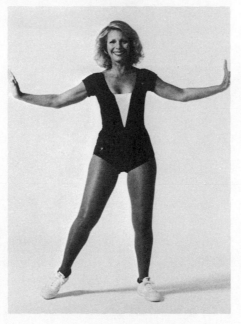
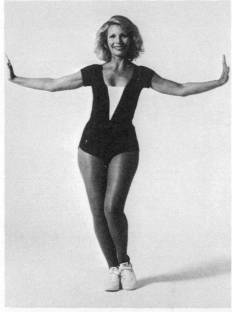

Begin with feet together, arms extended out at sides, shoulder height, with wrists flexed back, palms open and facing out. Step **right** with right foot as you smoothly rotate arms in a medium-sized circle, then

draw **left** foot in to right foot as you smoothly rotate arms in a second medium-sized circle.

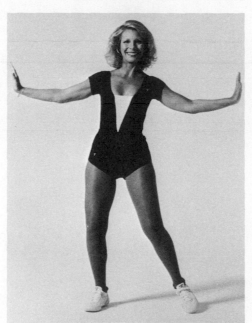
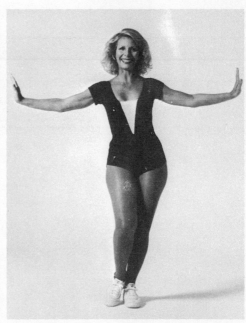

Step **left** with left foot as you smoothly rotate arms in a third circle, then

draw **right** foot in to left foot as you smoothly rotate arms in a fourth medium-sized circle.

1B. One-Step Arm Circles, Closed Down

*8 times forward; this takes
4 One-Steps
8 times backward; this takes
4 One-Steps*

Body benefits: strengthens and firms muscles in upper and lower arms and legs

Begin with feet together, arms extended out at sides, shoulder height, with hands in loose fists and dropped down from the wrists. Step **right** with right foot as you smoothly rotate arms in a medium-sized circle, then

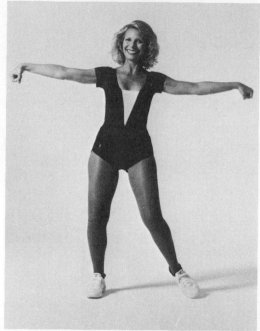 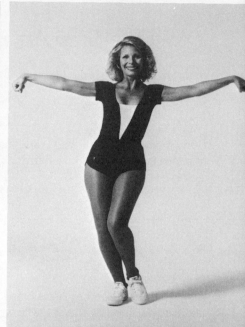

draw **left** foot in to right foot as you smoothly rotate arms in a second medium-sized circle.

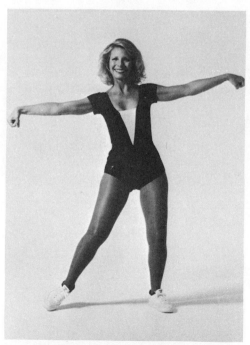 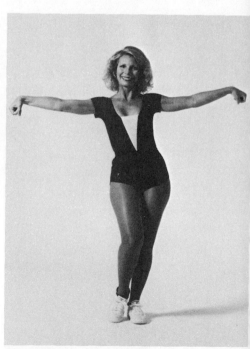

Step **left** with left foot as you smoothly rotate arms in a third circle, then

draw **right** foot in to left foot as you smoothly rotate arms in a fourth medium-sized circle.

2. One-Step Rope-Climbing

8 times, alternating right and left; this takes 8 One-Steps

Body benefits: strengthens arms, waist, sides of body and legs

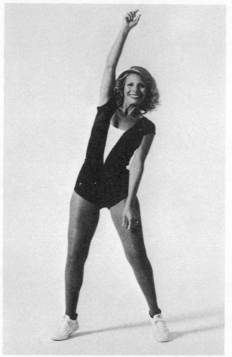

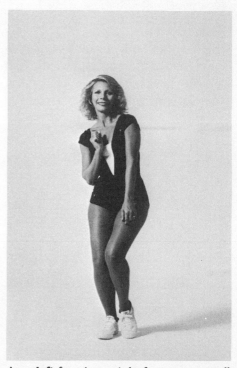

Begin with feet together, arms down in front with hands in loose fists. Step **right** with right foot as you reach right arm up overhead, then

draw **left** foot in to right foot as you pull right arm down.

THIS IS ONE TIME.

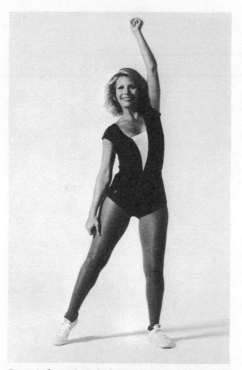

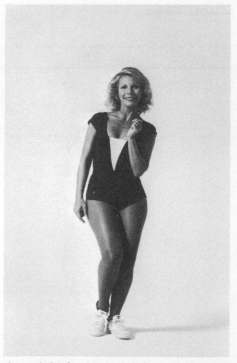

Step **left** with left foot as you reach left arm up overhead, then

draw **right** foot in to left foot as you pull left arm down.

3. One-Step Backstroke

8 times, alternating right and left; this takes 8 One-Steps

Body benefits: stretches arms, waist and sides of body, increases shoulder and lower back flexibility and strengthens legs

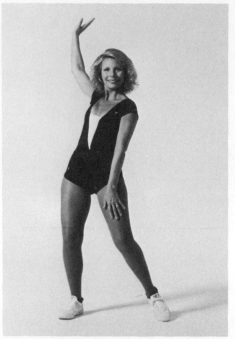 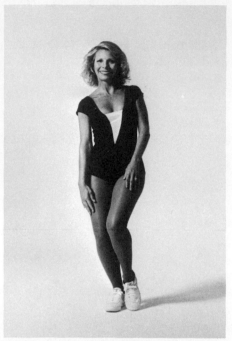

Begin with feet together, arms down in front, hands resting on front of thighs. Step **right** with right foot as you smoothly and continuously reach right arm forward and up, then

draw **left** foot in to right foot as you continue reaching around and down behind you and end with hand resting on front of right thigh.

THIS IS ONE TIME.

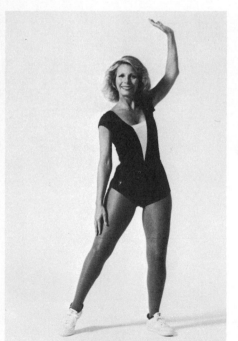 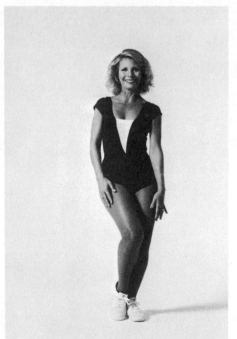

Step **left** with left foot as you smoothly and continuously reach left arm forward and up, then

draw **right** foot in to left foot as you continue reaching around and down behind you and end with hand resting on front of left thigh.

4. One-Step Snap-Down, Front

8 times; this takes 8 One-Steps

Body benefits: strengthens and firms arms, pectoral muscles and legs

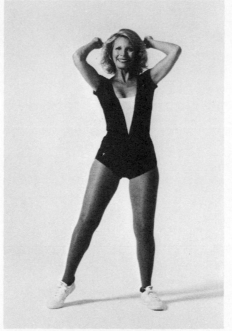

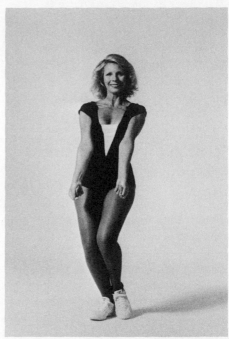

Begin with feet together, arms bent and held at your waist ("jogging arms"). Step **right** with right foot as elbows lift forward and move up in front of shoulders, hands in loose fists, then

draw **left** foot in to right foot as forearms extend forward and down, elbows straighten, and hands end with a snap of the fingers in front of thighs.

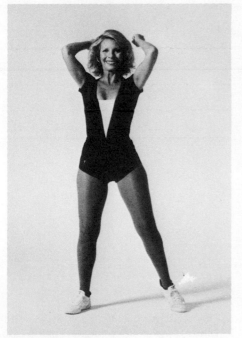

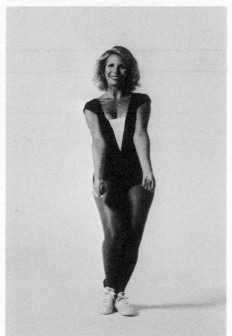

Step **left** with left foot as elbows move up in front of shoulders, hands in loose fists, then

draw **right** foot in to left foot as forearms extend forward and down and hands end with a snap of the fingers in front of thighs.

65

5. *One-Step Snap-Behind*

8 times; this takes 8 One-Steps

Body benefits: strengthens and firms arms, pectoral muscles and legs

Stand with your feet together, arms hanging at your sides.

Arms swing out at your sides to shoulder height as you step **right** with right foot. Hands are dropped down from wrists in loose fists, shoulders are back and down.

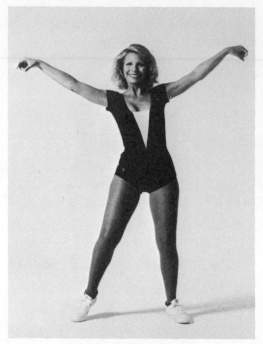 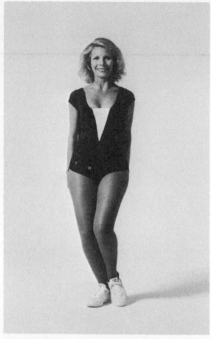

Draw **left** foot in to right foot as arms swing down at sides to end behind buttocks with a snap of your fingers.

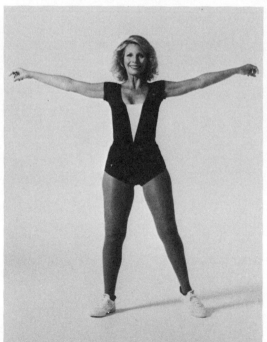 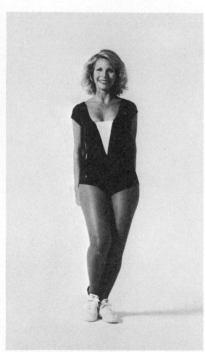

Step **left** with left foot as arms swing out at sides to end at shoulder level, then

draw **right** foot in to left foot as arms swing down at sides to end behind buttocks with a snap of your fingers.

6. One-Step Criss-Cross

4 counts low to high; this takes 4 One-Steps
4 counts high to low; this takes 4 One-Steps
4 counts low to high; this takes 4 One-Steps
4 counts high to low; this takes 4 One-Steps

Body benefits: stretches and firms arms and pectoral muscles and strengthens legs

Begin with feet together, arms extended down at sides, hands in loose fists.

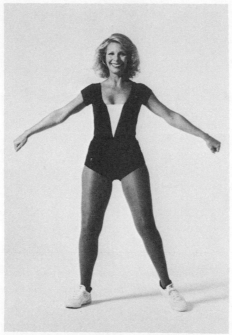

Count one: Step **right** with right foot as arms open in a wide "V" down in front of body, then

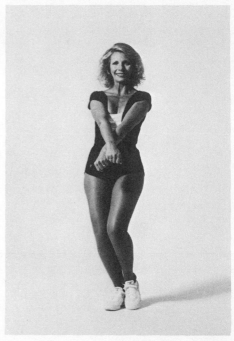

draw **left** foot in to right foot as you cross right arm over left arm at the lower arms, down in front of abdomen.

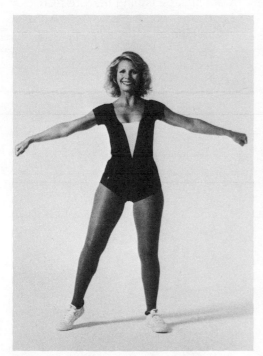

Count two: Step **left** with left foot as arms uncross to end extended in an open "V" in front of body at waist level, then

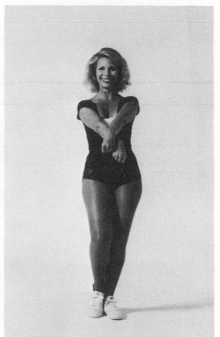

draw **right** foot in to left foot as you cross lower left arm over lower right arm at chest level.

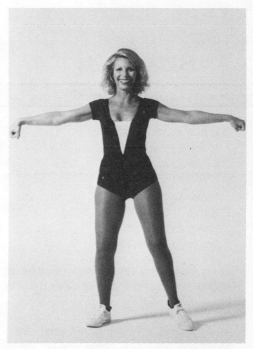

Count three: Step **right** with right foot as arms uncross to end extended in an open "V" in front of body at chest level, then

(continued)

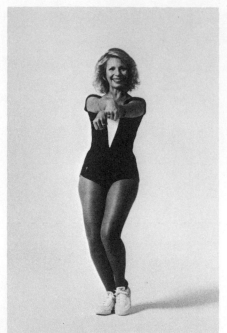

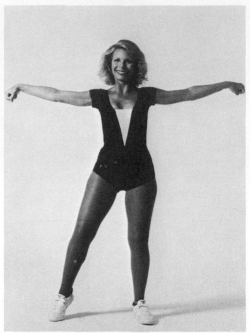

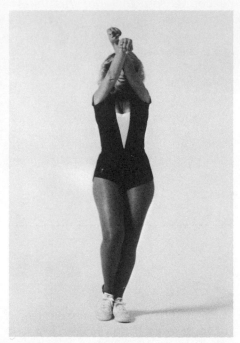

draw **left** foot in to right foot as you cross lower right arm over lower left arm at shoulder level.

Count four: Step **left** with left foot as arms uncross to end extended in an open "V" in front of body at shoulder level, then

draw **right** foot in to left foot as you cross lower left arm over lower right arm at head level.

Continue, beginning the Criss-Cross at head level, working down to low level in 4 One-Steps.

7. Side Bends

Do a total of 32, following this sequence:
8 times to the right
8 times to the left
4 times to the right
4 times to the left
2 times to the right
2 times to the left
2 times to the right
2 times to the left

Body benefits: stretches your waist and upper body, and increases flexibility in your lower back

Stand in stride position, left arm overhead and right arm down at side, hand resting loosely on thigh. Bend smoothly to the right keeping left arm on right thigh for support. Return to the upright position.

THIS IS ONE TIME TO THE RIGHT.

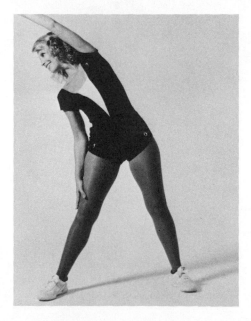

Repeat according to the pattern above, then reverse, bending to the left, and continue following pattern.

8. Twist and Snap

8 times, alternating right and left

Body benefits: stretches and firms upper body and increases flexibility in the lower back

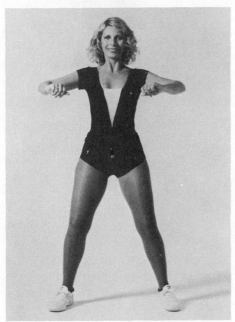

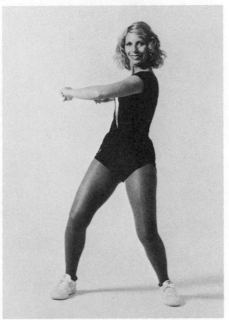

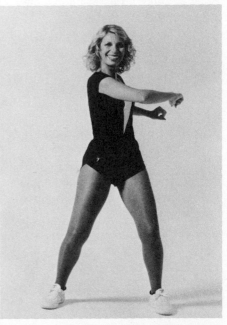

Stand in stride position, knees slightly bent, hands extended approximately 18″ in front of chest with elbows bent.

Smoothly twist arms and upper body to the right side with a snap of your fingers.

THIS IS ONE TIME.

Reverse, smoothly twisting arms, upper body and head to the left side with a snap of your fingers.

9. Jog, Low Level

8 sets of 8 jogging steps

Body benefits: aerobic!

Stand tall with abdominals pulled in and up.

Don't lean forward.

Land as much as possible on your full foot.

Whenever possible, *do not jog in place!* Instead, jog around the room or, better yet, in an interesting course around the house. This adds variety to your workout and puts less stress on your lower body.

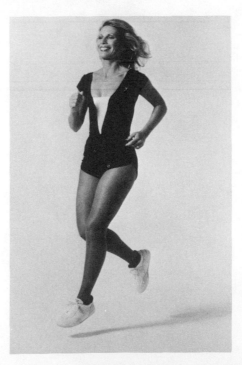

To make it easy to keep track of the number of jogs, clap your hands on the first count of each set of 8 and yell out the number of the set.

Clap and yell "One," then count to yourself 2-3-4-5-6-7-8 as you jog;

clap and yell "Two," then count to yourself 2-3-4-5-6-7-8 as you jog.

Continue until you've completed eight sets.

10. Knee-Lift Bounce Combo

Do 32 in this sequence:
8 times forward
8 times crossing
8 times forward
8 times open

Body benefits: front of thighs, back of thighs, and seat

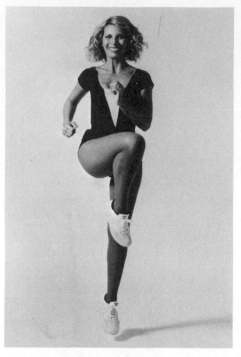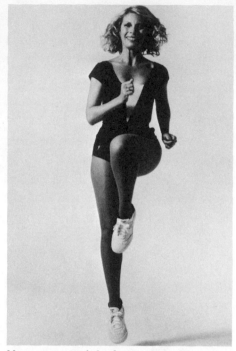

Knee-Lift Bounce, Forward—*8 times, alternating right and left*

Hop on your **left** foot as you lift your right knee up *in front,* then bounce **both feet** together.

THIS IS ONE TIME.

Hop on your **right** foot as you lift your left knee up *in front,* then bounce **both feet** together.

Knee-Lift Bounce, Crossing—*8 times, alternating right and left*

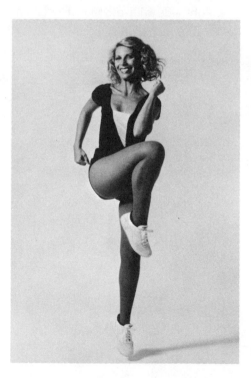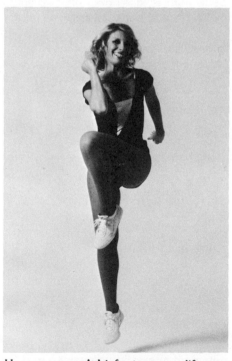

Hop on your **left** foot as you lift your right knee up *to point to left diagonal,* touch left elbow to knee, then bounce **both feet** together.

THIS IS ONE TIME.

Hop on your **right** foot as you lift your left knee up *to point to right diagonal,* touch right elbow to knee, then bounce **both feet** together.

Knee-Lift Bounce, Forward—*8 times, alternating right and left*

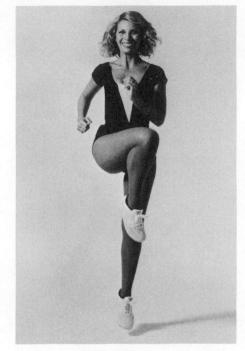

Hop on your **left** foot as you lift your right knee up *in front,* then bounce **both feet** together.

THIS IS ONE TIME.

Hop on your **right** foot as you lift your left knee up *in front,* then bounce **both feet** together.

Knee-Lift Bounce, Open—*8 times, alternating right and left*

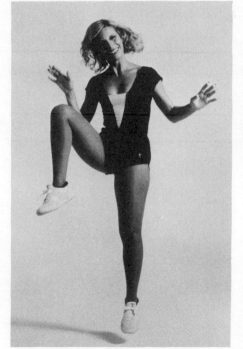

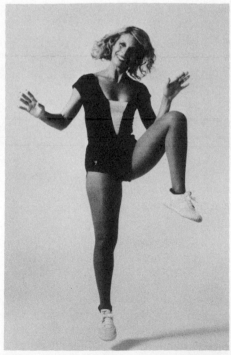

Hop on your **left** foot as you lift your right knee up *to point to the right diagonal,* hitting the top of your right thigh gently with your right hand, then bounce **both feet** together.

THIS IS ONE TIME.

Hop on your **right** foot as you lift your left knee up *to point to the left diagonal,* hitting the top of your left thigh gently with your left hand, then bounce **both feet** together.

71

11. Jog, Medium Level

8 sets of 8 jogging steps

Body benefits: aerobic!

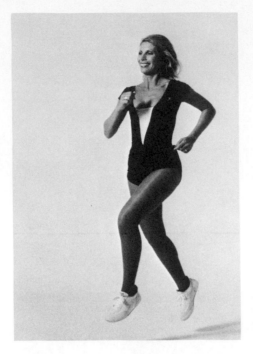

Lift your knees a little higher this time, and/or increase your speed.

Remember to keep your knees up in front and stand tall!

12. Kick-Jump Combo

Do 32 kick-jumps in this sequence:
8 forward
8 crossing
8 forward
8 open

Body benefits: legs, front of thighs, back of thighs, inner and outer thighs, and seat

Kick-Jump, Forward—*8 times, alternating right and left*

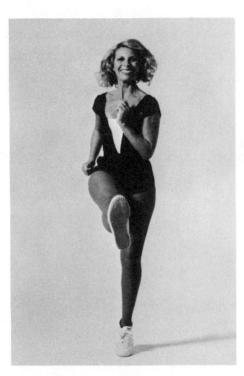

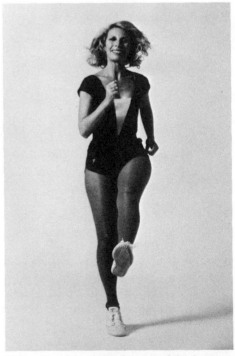

Hop on your **left** foot and kick your right foot *forward low* (no higher than waist level), then bounce **both feet** together.

THIS IS ONE TIME.

Hop on your **right** foot and kick your left foot *forward low* (no higher than waist level), then bounce **both feet** together.

72

Kick-Jump, Crossing—*8 times, alternating right and left*

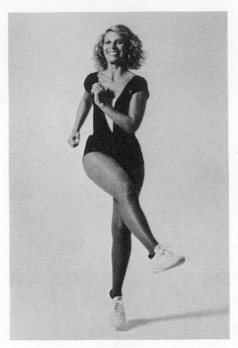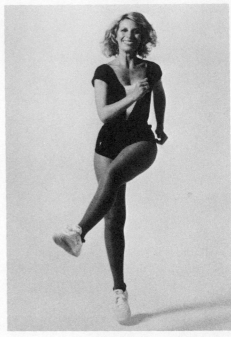

Hop on **left** foot and kick your right foot forward low *to the left diagonal* (no higher than waist level), then bounce **both feet** together.

THIS IS ONE TIME.

Hop on your **right** foot and kick your left foot forward low *to the right diagonal* (no higher than waist level), then bounce **both feet** together.

Kick-Jump, Forward—*8 times, alternating right and left*

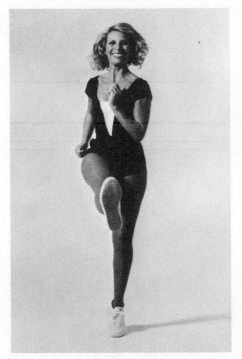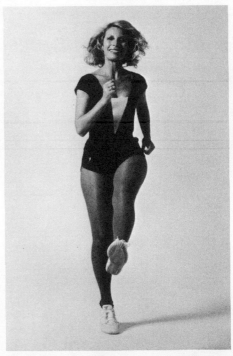

Hop on your **left** foot and kick your right foot *forward low* (no higher than waist level), then bounce **both feet** together.

THIS IS ONE TIME.

Hop on your **right** foot and kick your left foot *forward low* (no higher than waist level), then bounce **both feet** together.

(continued)

Kick-Jump Combo (continued)

Kick-Jump, Open—*8 times,*
alternating right and left

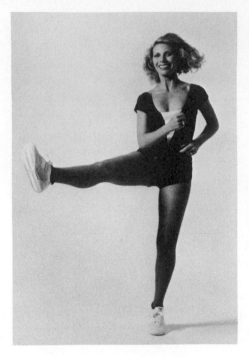
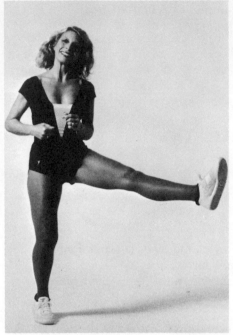

Hop on your **left** foot and kick your right
foot forward low *to the right diagonal*
(no higher than waist level), then
bounce **both feet** together.

THIS IS ONE TIME.

Hop on your **right** foot and kick your
left foot forward low *to the left diagonal*
(no higher than waist level), then
bounce **both feet** together.

13. *Jog, Medium Level*

8 sets of 8 jogging steps

Body benefits: aerobic!

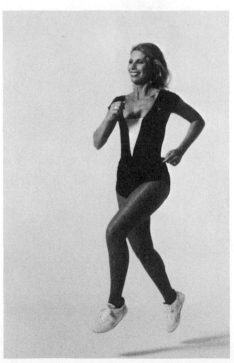

When you've finished this, you will have
jogged more than halfway around a
quarter-mile track! YEAH!

14. Rock Combo

Double Rock—*16 times, alternating right and left*
(This step takes 2 counts to each side and you should feel like the pendulum on a clock, swinging side to side.)

Body benefits: inner and outer thighs

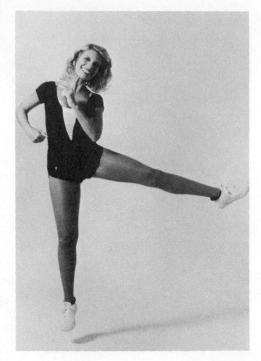

Rock to your **right** foot with right knee slightly bent and left leg extended out to the left side, then hop on your **right** foot—2 counts.

THIS IS ONE TIME. Then,

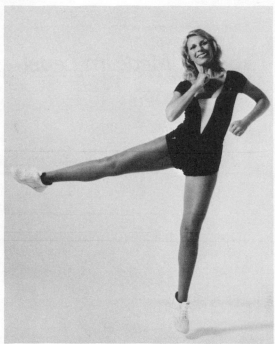

rock to your **left** foot with left knee slightly bent and right leg extended out to the right side, and hop on your **left** foot—2 counts.

(continued)

Rock Combo (continued)

Single Rock—*4 sets, 8 times each set, alternating right and left*
(This step takes 1 count to each side and is faster than the Double Rock because the hop is omitted)

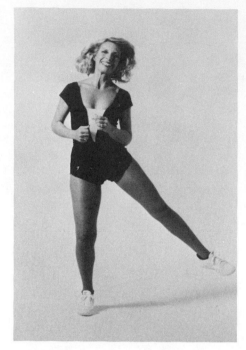

Rock to **right** foot with right knee slightly bent and left leg extended out to left side.

THIS IS ONE TIME. Then,

rock to **left** foot with left knee slightly bent and right leg extended out to right side.

15. *Jog, Medium Level*

8 sets of 8 jogging steps

Body benefits: aerobic!

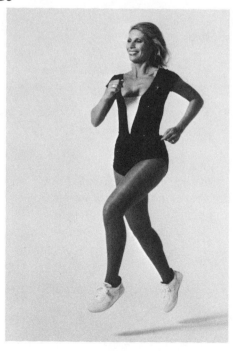
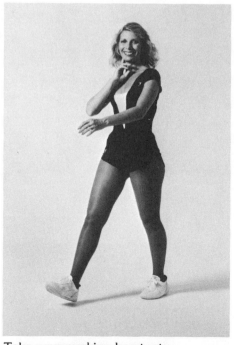

Lift your knees up in front.

Move mainly on the soles of your feet or flat-footed. Do not jog on your toes.

Maintain good posture and "jog tall."

Land lightly and don't stamp!

Take your working heart rate

NOTE: At this point, expand your aerobic benefits into a complete aerobic workout by going out for 15 to 20 minutes of jogging (approximately 8 laps around a track).

16. Cool-Down

Walk, Low Level—*8 sets of 8 steps*

You've now covered a quarter of a mile! Don't you feel GREAT?

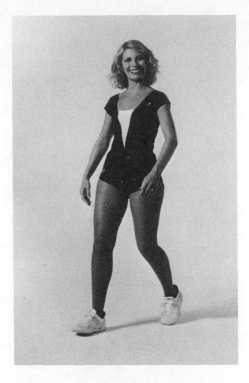

Calf Stretch—*8 slow counts for each leg*

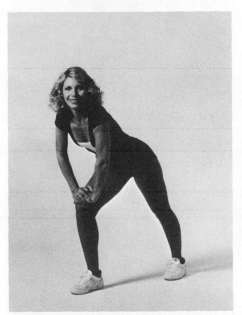

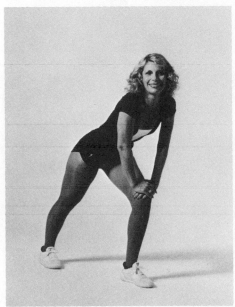

With feet together, keeping both feet pointing forward throughout, take a big step forward with **right** foot, bending right knee, keeping left leg straight. Place both hands above right knee with arms straight. Hold for 8 slow counts; then return to starting position.

Reverse stance, stepping forward with the **left** foot, left knee bent, right knee straight. Hands are placed above left knee. Hold for 8 slow counts, then return to starting position.

Take your recovery heart rate.

OPTIONAL ARM MOVEMENTS

Attention, both Brisk Walkers and Joggers! After you've been doing your Everyday Eights for a while and they're second nature, you may be interested in adding simple arm movements to your walking or jogging segments. This should be done gradually and progressively to make sure you are still staying within your individual working heart rate range. (Adding arm action will make your walking or jogging more aerobic, and therefore your working heart rate will be higher.)

Here are eight arm movements (for those of you who want to pretend you're an octopus. Ho ho!)

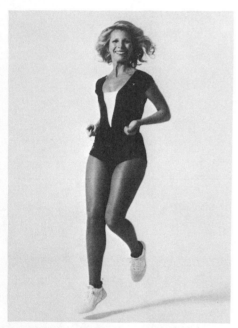

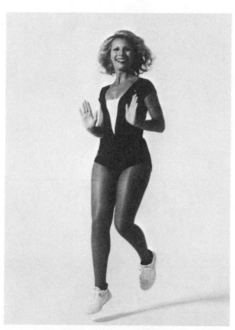

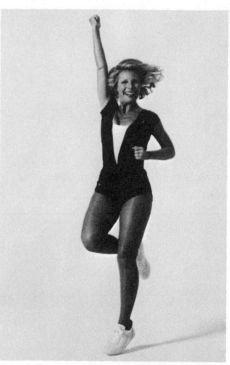

1. TWIRL: Keeping elbows close to waist and palms facing ceiling with hands in loose fists, circle lower arms and hands inward for each walking or jogging step. Pretend you're twirling two gold watches on chains.

2. SHINE: Keeping elbows close to waist and palms facing forward, circle lower arms and hands inward for each walking or jogging step. Pretend you're vigorously waxing and shining your car . . . use some elbow grease!

3. SINGLE WEIGHTS: With hands in loose fists and close in front of chest, lift one imaginary weight up overhead then pull it down for every two walking or jogging steps. Alternate right and left. You're Rocky and you're in weight training!

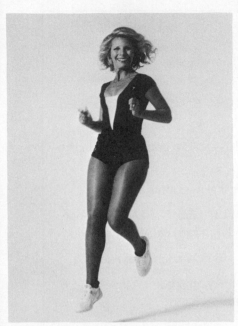 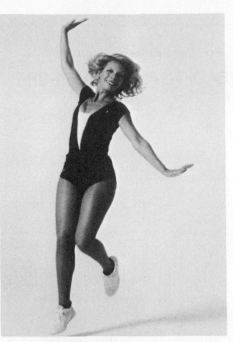 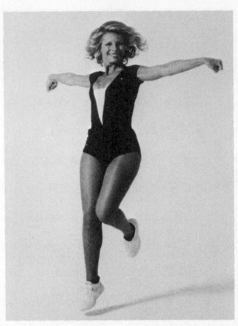

4. DRUMS: Keeping elbows close to waist and hands in loose fists, pretend you're playing the drums, alternating right and left, one beat for each walking or jogging step. Play the drums in all directions . . . you're part of a *jogging* marching band.

5. RAINBOWS: Stretch and circle right arm down and across body, up in front and around with palm out, ending down at right side for every four walking or jogging steps, then repeat with left arm. You're on vacation in Hawaii and get the thrill of seeing two rainbows at once!

6. PUNCH-OUT: Punch both arms out at sides then pull in for every 2 walking or jogging steps. Make room, world, here I come (once I get out of this sack)!

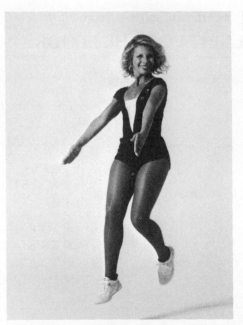 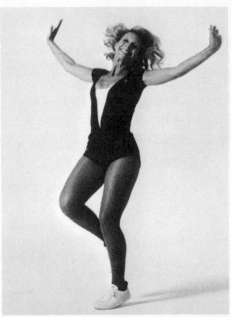

7. TRAIN: Keeping elbows close to waist and palms open facing sides of body, circle arms forward, down and around once for every 2 walking steps or jogs. It should look like the wheels moving on a locomotive. Time to jog on a different track . . . a *train* track.

8. SUNRISE: Stretch and circle both arms down, crossing in front, up and around with palms out, ending with arms extended out at sides for every four walking steps or jogs. This is my favorite because I feel as if I can touch the morning sky.

Everyday Eights—Segment I

HEAD-TO-TOE WARM-UP

1. SAY "NO"—8 times slowly

2. SAY "MAYBE"—8 times slowly

3. SAY "YES"—8 times slowly

4. SHOULDER ROLLS, SINGLE—8 times

5. SHOULDER ROLLS, DOUBLE—8 times

6. PULL-BACK STRETCH—8 times

7. SIDE BENDS—8 times

8. LOW BACK TWIST—8 times

9. KNEE-BEND STRETCH—8 times

10. SPORTY STRETCH—8 slow counts to each side

11. FLAMINGO FLING—8 slow counts for each leg

12. HAMSTRING STRETCH—2 times— Hold stretch for 8 slow counts each time

13. KNEE AND LOWER LEG STRETCH—4 outward circles and 4 inward circles for each leg

14. CALF STRETCH—8 slow counts for each leg

15. FOOT STRETCHES—4 outward circles and 4 inward circles for each foot

16. ON YOUR TOES—8 times

Everyday Eights—Segment II

EIGHT FOR THE FLOOR

1. STATIC STRETCH
   —To right leg, 8 slow counts
   —To left leg, 8 slow counts
   —Forward, 8 slow counts

2. KNEE PULL—8 times

3. LOWER BACK FLEXIBILITY ROLL—8 times

4. WRINGERS—8 times

5. SIDE LEG RAISERS
   —8 times with right leg, then roll to right side
   —8 times with left leg

6. THE CAT
   —8 times to the right, then knee in and down to floor
   —8 times to the left, then knee in and down to floor

7. LOW BACK STRETCH—hold stretch for 8 slow counts

8. SIT-UP TOUCH—8 times
   SIT-UP TWIST—8 times
   SIT-UP TOUCH—8 times
   SIT-UP TWIST—8 times

Everyday Eights—Segment III

TOP-TO-BOTTOM WORKOUT
(Brisk Walking Level)

1. ARM CIRCLES, PUSHED OUT
   —8 times forward
   —8 times backward

   ARM CIRCLES, CLOSED DOWN
   —8 times forward
   —8 times backward

2. ROPE-CLIMBING—8 times

3. BACKSTROKE—8 times

4. SNAP-DOWN, FRONT—8 times

5. SNAP-BEHIND—8 times

6. CRISS-CROSS
   —4 counts low to high
   —4 counts high to low
   —4 counts low to high
   —4 counts high to low

7. SIDE BENDS
   —8 times right; 8 times left
   —4 times right; 4 times left
   —2 times right; 2 times left
   —2 times right; 2 times left

8. TWIST AND SNAP—8 times

9. STROLL WALK—8 sets of 8 steps

10. KNEE-LIFT COMBO
    —Forward—8 times
    —Crossing—8 times
    —Forward—8 times
    —Open—8 times

11. BRISK WALK—8 sets of 8 steps

12. KICK COMBO
    —Forward—8 times
    —Crossing—8 times
    —Forward—8 times
    —Open—8 times

13. BRISK WALK—8 sets of 8 steps

14. SIDE LEG-LIFTS—16 times

15. BRISK WALK—8 sets of 8 steps
    —WORKING HEART RATE
    —NOTE: At this point, expand your aerobic benefits into a complete aerobic workout by taking a 30-minute walk (approximately 8 laps around a track).

16. COOL-DOWN
    —Stroll Walk—8 sets of 8 steps
    —Calf Stretch—8 slow counts for each leg
    —RECOVERY HEART RATE

TOP-TO-BOTTOM WORKOUT
(Jogging Level)

1. ONE-STEP ARM CIRCLES, PUSHED OUT
   —8 times forward
   —8 times backward
   ONE-STEP ARM CIRCLES, CLOSED DOWN
   —8 times forward
   —8 times backward

2. ONE-STEP ROPE-CLIMBING—8 times

3. ONE-STEP BACKSTROKE—8 times

4. ONE-STEP SNAP-DOWN, FRONT—8 times

5. ONE-STEP SNAP-BEHIND—8 times

6. ONE-STEP CRISS-CROSS
   —4 counts low to high
   —4 counts high to low
   —4 counts low to high
   —4 counts high to low

7. SIDE BENDS
   —8 times right; 8 times left
   —4 times right; 4 times left
   —2 times right; 2 times left
   —2 times right; 2 times left

8. TWIST AND SNAP—8 times

9. JOG, LOW LEVEL—8 sets of 8 jogging steps

10. KNEE-LIFT BOUNCE COMBO
    —Forward—8 times
    —Crossing—8 times
    —Forward—8 times
    —Open—8 times

11. JOG, MEDIUM LEVEL—8 sets of 8 jogging steps

12. KICK-JUMP COMBO
    —Forward—8 times
    —Crossing—8 times
    —Forward—8 times
    —Open—8 times

13. JOG, MEDIUM LEVEL—8 sets of 8 jogging steps

14. ROCK COMBO
    —Double Rock—16 times
    —Single Rock—4 sets of 8

15. JOG, MEDIUM LEVEL
    —8 sets of 8 jogging steps
    —WORKING HEART RATE!
    —NOTE: At this point, expand your aerobic benefits into a complete aerobic workout by going out for 15 to 20 minutes of jogging (approximately 8 laps around a track).

16. COOL-DOWN
    —Walk—8 sets of 8 steps
    —Calf Stretch—8 slow counts for each leg
    —RECOVERY HEART RATE

3

Whistle, Whistle, Let's Go!

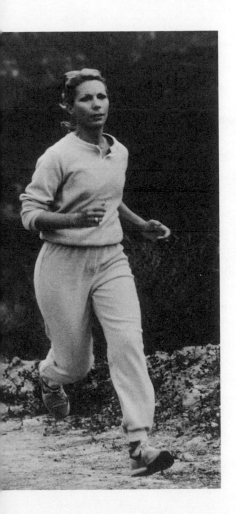

In 1971, jogging wasn't popular and aerobic exercise opportunities for women were limited. This led me to develop Aerobic Dancing, a program that catered almost exclusively to women who were physically inactive and wanted an effective way to shape up that would be fun to do.

Since then, hundreds of thousands of women and men have been motivated to keep coming back for one 12-week session after another. During this time, I've been encouraging my students to add a third and fourth day of aerobic activity to their life every week. Some of them take a third day of Aerobic Dancing while many others have added new aerobic activities.

In the meantime, this country has experienced the running phenomenon, the tennis and racquetball booms, and even a revival of roller skating. Now I have people coming into my program who are already fit, but who want to enjoy moving in a greater variety of ways. Either it's inconvenient for them to participate three or four times a week in one activity, or they tell me, "I'm a runner, but I'm only running two days a week now because I want to do something different and I want to use my upper body more." So they devote two days a week to Aerobic Dancing and two days to running. This is great because there's a smorgasbord of aerobic activities to choose from that can add pleasure to anyone's fitness program.

I like to talk in terms of minimums. When it comes to achieving minimum aerobic fitness, you should participate in some type of aerobic exercise at least twice a week on non-consecutive days and devote at least 30 minutes to each workout (including your warm-up and cool-down). By participating twice a week, you're going to begin to enjoy fitness benefits all over. You should notice inches leave your body while you gain more daily energy.

Once you've adjusted to this weekly pattern and you're experiencing these benefits, you'll be motivated to add a third aerobic workout each week: a fitness walk, racquetball, cycling, or perhaps swimming. And, with a little extra planning at home or at work, you can easily manage a fourth day. With a positive attitude, fitness can become play and you'll soon be saying, "Look at all the fun I've been missing!"

Four aerobic workouts a week is your goal. You should find a basic activity that you like well enough to do two times a week without fail. Call this your "core" aerobic program—walking, jogging, Aerobic Dancing, or whatever. You may simply want to do this one activity or sport four times a week, but why not explore other aerobic activities? With the improved muscle tone, increased self-confidence, and new-found energy you've gained from your core program, you can go out and enjoy many new fitness experiences.

> Some people like that downhill stuff
> They like it fast and breezy
> Some people walk on the other side
> They like it slow and easy.
>
> Some people run on a mountain trail
> Some like it wild and rough
> Some like to fly and some like to sail
> Some like the downhill stuff.
>
> But whatever we do
> We gotta do our own thing!

So don't be afraid to experiment. You're a winner each time you go out and try!

Another motivating reason to expand your fitness horizons is to prevent injuries. As we grow older, it becomes increasingly important to balance activities that are weight-bearing, such as jogging, tennis, or Aerobic Dancing, with non—weight-bearing endeavors such as cycling, swimming, and walking. This diversity will enable you to balance the stress placed on specific joints and bones, use your muscles in different ways, and help prevent your "burning-out" from too much of one sport or fitness pursuit.

Up until 1977 I kept fit by running 30 to 40 miles a week and dancing up to 16 hours a week. I had had a couple of injuries, and I started thinking, If you really want to keep running and dancing in the years to come, you have to exercise *some* degree of moderation. So I started investigating other sports and activities that I felt I might enjoy trying. Since then I've cut back on my running, and I now do half my dancing at a jogging level and half at a running level. Also, I use stationary cycling, swimming, and walking to round out my fitness week.

Here then are the aerobic activities I suit up for because they fit *my* lifestyle:

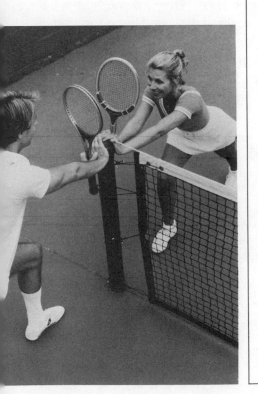

INJURY PREVENTION SAFEGUARDS

• Whatever aerobic activity you choose to do, remember to always WARM UP slowly with flexibility exercises before you begin and COOL DOWN afterwards with walking and calf stretches. These are universal safety factors that apply to any sport or exercise program. Remember, too, that a young body can take almost anything, but as you grow older, warming up and cooling down properly become increasingly important to your body's well-being, your performance, and your enjoyment of that activity.

• If you want a flexibility and stretching routine that will prepare you for almost any aerobic activity, just use the five-minute Head-to-Toe Warm-up in my Everyday Eights workout. Don't overlook this even for non–weight-bearing exercises such as swimming or cycling.

• An effective fitness activity should help relieve tension and stress from your life, so *relax your mind* as you get warmed up and ready to dance, exercise, or play a sport.

• Tight calf muscles can lead to shinsplints or other muscle pulls, which is why I'm adamant about calf stretches at the end of each Aerobic Dancing class. Make them an integral part of any workout.

• Give your feet a little breather at the end of a vigorous aerobic activity by untying your shoelaces and retying them loosely.

• If you're starting a new aerobic activity (particularly from a sedentary life-style) remember that it's easy—and dangerous—to fall into the "too much, too soon, too fast" syndrome. Jumping into a new activity without practicing the principle of gradual progression nearly always results in sore, aching muscles and perhaps even an injury. This leads to a natural inclination (and "justification") to want to drop out.

• If you take a break from your established aerobic activity for more than a week or two, it's equally important to start gradually and progressively when you return. I know this is a challenge when you're proficient in an activity, but you must take this precaution.

• One of the common signs that you've over-exerted in any aerobic activity is when you feel unusually tired or sleepy about two hours after the end of the workout. If this happens to you, exercise less vigorously next time. Other indications of overexertion are an overly flushed face, slight dizziness, and a feeling of nausea.

JOGGING/RUNNING

Running has been a vital part of my lifestyle since 1970, when I started training for my first (and only) marathon. This was back when few women were distance runners and I wanted to prove to myself that I could finish a marathon by training through a combination of running and Aerobic Dancing.

I trained over a year for that race in Atlantic City, running 20-plus miles a week and dancing 25 hours (my Aerobic Dancing program was just getting under way and I was doing all of the teaching). When the race came, there were exactly three women in the field, hard as that might be to imagine today. It was the physical challenge of my life trying to finish 26 miles, 385 yards, but I didn't want to have invested all those miles and weeks of training for nothing. I'm not a competitive person in sports, but I'm extremely competitive with myself; when I start something, I stick with it until I finish it.

So, I completed my marathon on October 24, 1971 (3 hours; 35 minutes), and I've been celebrating that date every year since then—celebrating the fact that I have not run a marathon again! I applaud marathoners, but running that distance just isn't *my* idea of an enjoyable *recurring* experience. As soon as I finished the Atlantic City race, I felt I had climbed my Mount Everest and once was enough. I was also burned out. When I came home, I thought, "Well, you've done it—what's left?" I realized that I had been running for the marathon as an end in itself—not for fitness or for fun. I stopped running for about three months, but then I gradually took it up again, this time for enjoyment. I wasn't training for anything, I wasn't recording my mileage, and I gradually learned to love running again.

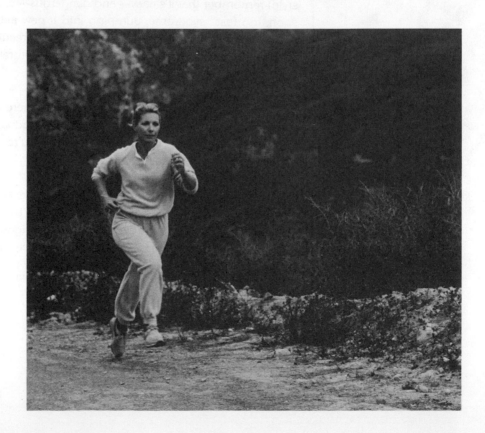

One personal change I've noticed over the years is that when I first started running, I often had to play mental games to keep going. If I felt like stopping the run before I had reached my distance goal or time goal, I'd say, "Just one more minute . . . or one more lap . . . or one more block, and then I'll see how I feel." Now when I run 30 to 40 minutes (and occasionally one hour) I don't even think of how far or how fast I'm going because *how long I last* is the key, and that's how I set my pace. What researchers are now finding is that it's better to keep going longer—and last—than it is to go too fast and have to stop.

When running, I enjoy letting my mind flow free, and by doing this I have at times come up with solutions to business challenges or choreography blocks. I'll even abruptly stop running to try out a new step or transition in the middle of my running route. It's dull to *appear* too sane!

Running Hints:

1. Invest in a great pair of running shoes, and don't run in worn-out shoes.

2. Buy "waffle" soles if you run on grassy or dirt surfaces and "ripple" soles for pavement running.

3. The best running advice I ever received was this: "run full-footed with a gentle heel-to-toe motion."

4. Run lightly, not only by landing gently but by "striding tall," by keeping your abdominals pulled in and up, and by using your arms in a mildly vigorous way so they help carry the load.

5. Vary your running routes, for there's so little time . . . and so much to see!

*Got the sun in my eyes
and the wind in my face
and it's good just to be alive!*

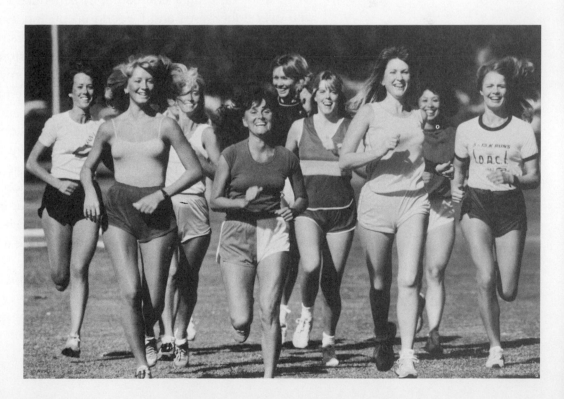

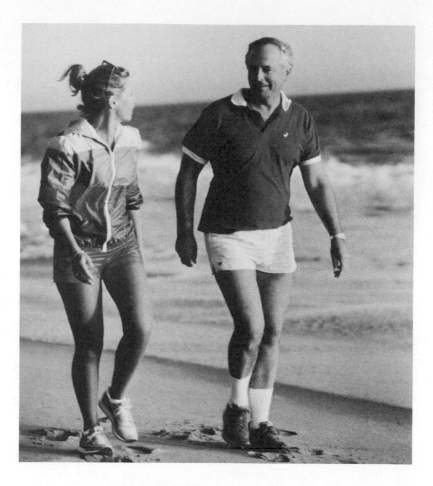

WALKING

Once while on a tight choreography schedule, I went for two or three days with over-tight calves and I wound up pulling a hamstring muscle. I hadn't increased my calf stretching to balance the increased dancing load. So, I learned a good lesson about the value of calf stretches but I also discovered the joys—and virtues—of brisk walking during my recovery period.

Neil and I now use walking to help improve our lifestyle in several ways. We walk together every night, catching up on each other's day. We're away from the television, telephone, and the temptation to sit down for the rest of the evening. When Neil comes home, he's hungry but instead of snacking—which was his custom a few years ago—he quickly changes and we do the Everyday Eights workout. Then we leave the house to continue our aerobic workout. Sometimes we walk briskly for an hour in our neighborhood, or we drive down the hill and really step out along the beach. At least three times a week we head for the local running track, where we run for 30 to 40 minutes and finish up the hour by walking.

In Aerobic Dancing, I've come up with several types of walks for pacing purposes, but Neil and I do the Fitness Walk or the Talk Walk—which is walking as fast as you can while talking as fast as you can to your partner. Our plan is to always end up with an hour of combined jog/walk action whatever we do, and that's *in addition* to the Everyday Eights and our calf-stretch cool-down.

Walking Hints

1. Not only is walking an excellent way to get in shape, and stay in shape, but I'm now keenly aware of just how effective it is as a *fat-burning* activity. Researchers tell us that although the "after-exercise calorie-burn" effect lasts longer with one continuous walk (a minimum of 15 to 20 minutes), you can walk an hour a day by doing it in short segments and still get most of the same fat-burning benefits.

2. Do you catch yourself saying, "Gee, I never have enough time to really talk to my kids or to my husband"? If so, how about working family walks into your schedule, like right after dinner before everybody settles into the nightly routine? I know fathers, for example, who try to take their kids with them on a walk to the store. They leave the car at home and they spend the time with their kids talking and getting exercise together, while also taking care of errands. That's the get-it-all-together approach I love to see!

3. Another reason walking has recently gained such popularity as a wonderful aerobic workout is the growing awareness that the length of your workout is more important than its intensity. Most people can walk longer than they can jog or run (while absorbing less weight-bearing stress on the body in the process). There's also the back-to-nature aspect of walking that is shared by runners. I'll never forget a special morning walk when I spotted a lively lizard, four species of butterflies, and some pink flowers as tiny as a tear while doing my calf stretches. What rewards!

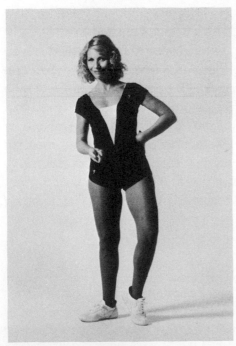

Charlie Chaplin Walk

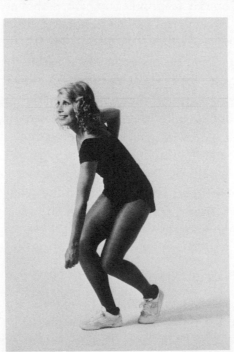

Camel Walk

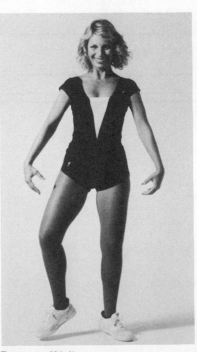

Penguin Walk

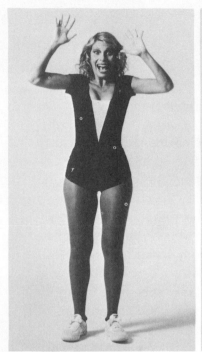
E.T.-Meets-Gertie Walk

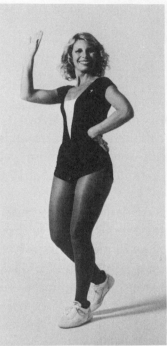
Rose Parade Walk

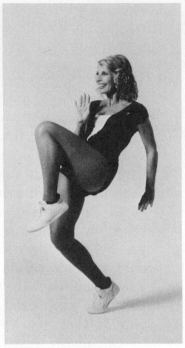
Truckin' Walk

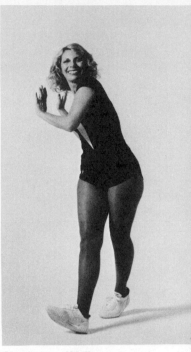
Charleston Walk

RIDING A STATIONARY BIKE

Contrary to popular opinion, stationary cycling *does* get you somewhere and it doesn't have to be boring. So come on—give the stationary bike another chance! (Especially if you already have one that stands unused.)

To motivate yourself, find something to keep your mind occupied as you cycle. Pretend you're pumping away the miles on a fantasy airborne bike trip across the moon as you listen to the soundtrack from the movie *E.T.* Watch your favorite television show, listen to Books on Tape, or catch up on that ever-growing stack of reading material. I find that if I'm on the phone or reading, I forget I'm pedaling. Also, this bike activity means more to me than keeping fit. I'm a get-it-all-together person because I want to do so much every day. Thus, getting on the bike gives me a chance to learn and grow, whether it's a book I'm reading or a videotape I'm watching. This is how *I* learned to love my bike.

Biking Hints:

1. Get a cushioned seat cover for a more comfortable ride, or fold a bath towel in half for extra seat softness.

2. Invest in a reading-rack attachment so you don't get your reading material sweaty.

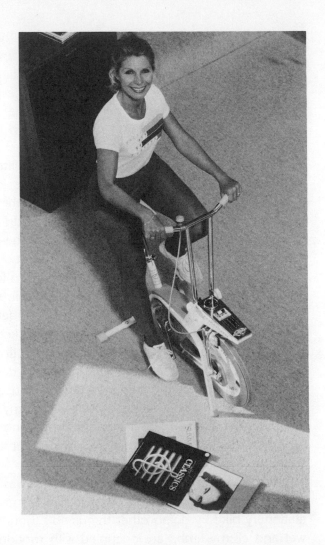

3. Place your whole sole on the pedal, not just your toes.

4. Your legs should almost fully extend on each revolution without shifting your body side to side and without raising your heels.

5. After warming up, begin by cycling at a low tension setting for five minutes, then gradually increase the tension to a point where you're getting a workout that's still enjoyable.

6. Before dismounting, gradually decrease the tension as you continue cycling at a relaxed level and begin to cool down.

SWIMMING

I started using our back-yard swimming pool for exercise in 1977. It was summer and I wanted a new aerobic activity I could do outside. I don't particularly enjoy getting my face in the water, but I love the clean, cool rush of water over my body, so I thought I'd give swimming a try—my way.

The first day I thought, Let's see how long I can last doing the sidestroke. This is my favorite stroke and I wanted to be gentle with myself, which is the approach I always advocate when trying something new. Well, ten minutes is all I lasted. My arms and legs were like lead and I was huffing and puffing, even though I was in excellent dry-land condition. My first reaction was, This is ridiculous; I'll swim for fun but not for fitness. Then I started thinking, It must be an incredible workout if I feel like this after ten minutes—I'll bet I was also tense and not breathing properly. Then I thought, I'll try for *twelve* minutes tomorrow. The challenge was on!

The next day I pushed myself and I lasted fifteen minutes before I got that same worked-out feeling. It took me four weeks to work up to an hour of swimming (with a five-minute break halfway through), which is a fairly rapid progression, but I was fit when I started and I'm a fast learner on how to streamline effort. Even though I reached the one-hour plateau within a month, *it wasn't a goal.* My plan was to simply take it one lap at a time and see how I felt. If somebody had told me, "You can swim for fitness but it has to be the Australian crawl done a minimum of thirty minutes or you're never going to get any benefit," then I would have said, "Forget it," and I would never have experienced the fluid sensation of a water workout.

Once I discovered I could handle one continuous hour in the pool doing the sidestroke, that challenge was met and I decided to simply concentrate on a continuous thirty-minute workout because it was more enjoyable. Instead of counting laps—a deadly trap—I put my kitchen timer by the edge of the pool. Once again, the important thing is not the vigor or the number of laps you're able to complete in swimming, but the length of time that you're in the pool *moving.*

An obvious challenge I had to overcome was boredom, because you can only think so much as you swim. I had learned to cope with this on the stationary bike by doing other things so I thought, What can I do when I'm wet and all my limbs are occupied with motion? The perfect solution was music!

When I want to mentally relax, I play classical records. At times music is for thought, and I feel the better the music the better the thoughts. By swimming the sidestroke, I can also look up at the sky and see the clouds, the hummingbirds, and even the wasps who alight for a quick drink. Seeing all these wondrous things is a relaxing, stress-reducing experience.

If I want to "work" as I swim, I listen to records I'm screening for choreography. When I hear a good song, I jump out of the pool, go over to my pad on the patio table, and jot down the name of the song and my ideas for a possible dance. Then I dive back in and resume swimming. This adds variety to my swim and I get more done.

Swimming Hints:

1. Swimming is a fluid exercise (pun intended) and perhaps your body can function safely without a warm-up, but it has been my experience—and it makes sense—to prepare yourself from head to toe.

2. After a swimming workout you need five minutes of walking and calf stretching, I feel, before you sit down.

3. If I've encouraged you to try swimming for fitness because the side-stroke sounds do-able, you can protect your hair and face from the sun by wearing sun block and a baseball hat as I do.

4. Each time I make a turn in the pool, I switch arms for a more balanced workout. It wasn't easy at first, but it's one of the tricks I use to last longer. (Of course, this only applies to the sidestroke.)

5. When I run and swim on the same day, I always swim last because it soothes my feet.

6. On vacations at the beach I try to find a sheltered area with little or no surf so I can swim up and down the shoreline instead of out and back. When I switch sides I get a new view!

7. Simple exercises become even more beneficial when done in a pool with the added resistance of the water. Here are three examples of how to take my Aerobic Dancing steps into the pool:

One-Step Backstroke

Do a One-Step as seen on page 60 and Backstroke arms as seen on page 48.

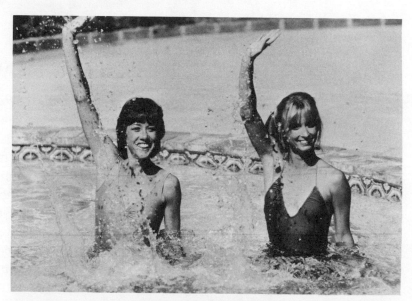

Breast Stroke

Begin with feet in wide stride position, hands close in front of chest, palms open. Bend right knee as body sways right and arms push forward and around through the water. Bend left knee as body sways left and arms continue around to end close in front of chest. Reverse directions to breast-stroke left.

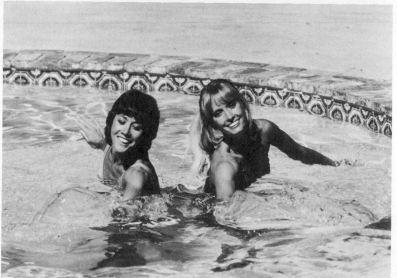

Knee-Lift Step, with Lift Arms

Begin with feet together, arms down at sides. Lift right knee as high as is comfortable, as left arm lifts up in front to overhead and right arm lifts up in back to overhead. Step **right** foot next to left foot as arms return down to sides. Reverse, lifting left knee and lifting right arm up in front and left arm up in back.

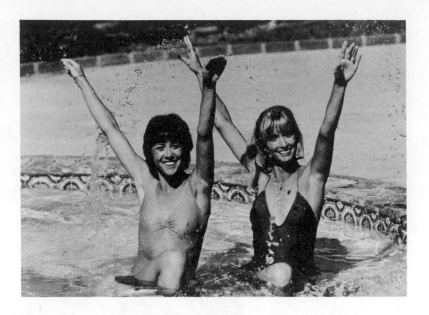

TENNIS (PLAYED AEROBICALLY)

Normally, I wouldn't list tennis as an *aerobic* activity, but lately Neil and I have been playing more often during the year—not simply on our summer vacation—so I *sometimes* add extra touches in order to gain an aerobic workout.

First of all, I jog to retrieve balls on my side of the net, and I jog back into position to start the next point. I sometimes even jog in place as I wait for Neil to serve and I run to the other end of the court when we change sides. All this extra effort burns more calories and keeps my heart rate at an aerobic level for a longer period of time. If all this sounds a bit too energetic for your tastes (or physical conditioning), then just gradually make some adjustments—like jogging to retrieve every other ball at the net. Or just play for recreation—I love doing that too.

This isn't to downplay or overlook the physical benefits of this game, such as the aerobic and calorie-burning results that a good, solid hour of singles play can yield, the continual stretching and bending to hit the ball, and the upper-body action used when serving properly.

Tennis Hints:

1. In a stop-and-start sport like tennis, you're stretching your luck if you don't do your stretches beforehand. This is especially true for your lower back and upper body. Also make sure you get your serving arm warmed up and your shoulder loose by first going through the service motion without the racquet. Then take imaginary serves with the racquet, but without a ball.

2. Make sure your feet are adequately supported in all directions by wearing proper foot gear.

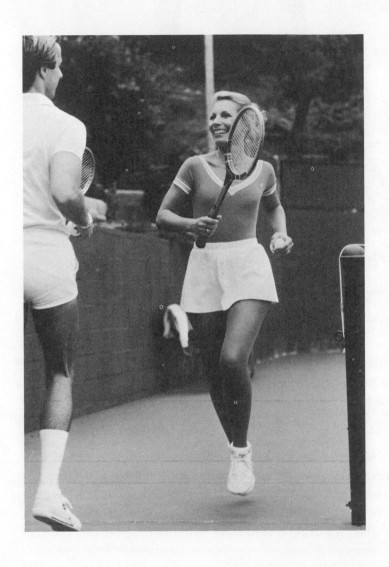

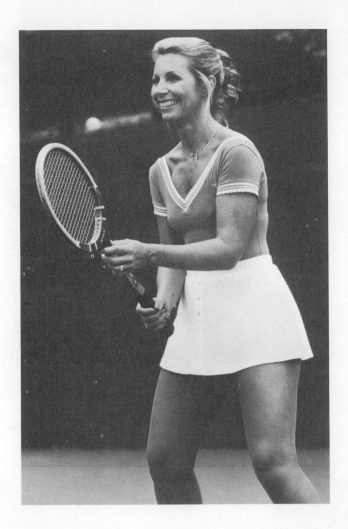

3. Don't try to hit out-of-bounds balls. You may stretch beyond your own bounds and end up with an ache or a pain.

4. When you double fault or miss an overhead smash, don't break your racquet over your knee. This could lead to painful bruises.

OTHER AEROBIC ACTIVITIES

There are a number of other excellent aerobic activities that you might already be enjoying. They aren't a regular part of my lifestyle at the moment, but I'm hoping some of them will be in the next few years, at least seasonally or when I travel.

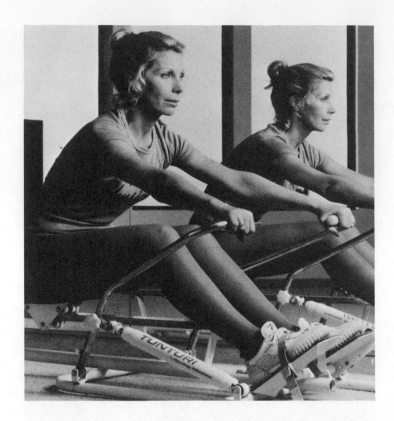

- **Rowing.** I'm finding my new rowing machine to be an interesting way to work out my upper body on non–Aerobic Dancing days and get an aerobic workout at the same time. I was a crew fan in college so now I pretend I'm on the team!

- **Riding a bike.** Neil and I no longer ride our bikes because we live in an area where it's easier to do other things, but what fun we have when we're in New York City on a weekend and we can ride the six-mile loop around Central Park. If you enjoy riding a bike, did you know that you can turn your outdoor bike into an indoor bike by buying a simple attachment?

- **Cross-country skiing.** I tried it once and loved it, and if I had the time I'd be out there doing it every winter . . . so I'll follow my own advice and make the time!

- **Racquetball.** This is a highly rated conditioner and certainly a vigorous outlet for your competitive impulses. Now to find a friend who's patient enough to teach me!

- If your community has a **par course** exercise circuit, this can be a great way to participate by yourself, with your family, or with friends.

- **Jumping rope.** I've temporarily given this up as an aerobic activity, because I'm concentrating on Aerobic Dancing and running and tennis as my weight-bearing activities for the time being. However, if you love to skip rope and it's a gratifying activity for you (not too many misses), then jump to it! It will always be one of my favorite indoor activities.

MAINTAINING YOUR FITNESS PROGRAM

Planning, flexibility, and spontaneity are all equally important when it comes to maintaining a sensible fitness program that inspires you day to day, week to week, and season to season.

Again, the basic aerobic system I recommend is to strive for 20 to 30 minutes of continuous aerobic activity four times a week. Ideally, plan and program yourself two times a week—utilizing your favorite activity—and be *spontaneous* two times a week. With experience it becomes easy to follow your own instincts and personal preferences as the year goes along, perhaps shifting from skiing and ice skating in the winter to long hikes and bike rides in the summer. This variety and moderation will keep you enthusiastic about your opportunities to keep fit, and should help you avoid becoming an exercise dropout. Some people simply add stress to their lives by forcing themselves to pursue physical fitness as yet another duty. I feel that negative motivation like this rarely works over the long haul. Remember: you can't store fitness, you can only store fat, so your love for fitness must be endless —and it *will* be when you find aerobic experiences that give you a lift!

Although you may find that it helps to set specific long-range fitness goals, a week-by-week, or even a day-by-day approach is enough if you stick with it. When I was training for the marathon, I felt it was important to keep careful records of my aerobic activity, since I was following Dr. Kenneth Cooper's point system and I was determined to have my body prepared to handle 26 miles (and 385 yards!). Reviewing my training diary also provided an important incentive to spur me on. Yet once the race was over, I realized that my training experience had enabled me to sense what my body needed and what it meant to be fit. I found that I could plan my exercise one day at a time because I knew intuitively if I was getting enough vigorous activity during the day to maintain my high level of fitness.

This isn't to say that it's unnecessary to record *your* aerobic efforts from day to day. You may find, as I did, that a journal can provide a warm feeling of success. Writing everything down and then seeing that you can stick with your program week after week is inspiring!

These days, I get up, have my breakfast, and then take a look at my schedule and determine how and when I'm going to get my fitness breaks. That's as important to me as fulfilling my different business commitments. If I'm going to have a photography session all afternoon, then I know that I absolutely need one hour of exercise beforehand in order to be ready mentally, emotionally, and physically for that challenge. Generally I dance or I go out for a walk. If I'm faced with a day of writing against deadlines, "must" reading, and business meetings, I'll try to work in two to three hours of exercise, evenly spaced through the day. By having a plan like this, even the most high-tension days are balanced by physical outlets that enable me to work happily and efficiently.

Another way to build in extra motivation is to find an equally committed partner. What really helps me get my second or third hour of aerobic activity every day is having somebody like Neil to exercise with. Neil, too, admits that he'd be less likely to go out for a walk/run by himself if he came home from work and I had already had my quota of exercise for the day. So we help motivate each other.

This helps explain why many group exercise programs are so popular. If you enroll in a course with a friend—or run every other day with a friend—there'll be days when you're "down" but your friend is "up" and gets you going. Or, when your friend is down, there's a chance you'll be up. So encourage your friends (or family members) to join you in your exercise activities . . . especially walking. You can walk and talk instead of calling each other on the phone. (If you're looking for time to spend with your spouse or other family members, why not get involved together in a fitness activity?)

Even with the best of intentions to always stick to your fitness program, there are going to be days and weeks when you simply can't find the time or motivation. My advice is to have the attitude that you're going to make exercise a part of every day, like brushing your teeth and eating. You *always* fit those things in, right? On some days, it's true, you have to just *do your fitness.* Don't expect it to be a thrill or a glorious experience, but don't make it negative—just *DO IT!* Believe me, there are days when I don't even want to go out for a walk, let alone a run, but I still go out with Neil because I know I'll feel better, . . . and it works!

SELECTING AN EXERCISE PROGRAM THAT MEETS YOUR NEEDS

With the multitude and variety of exercise programs available today, I felt it would be helpful to provide you with a checklist of questions to ask before joining exercise classes that feature "aerobics." You deserve to know that you're investing your time and money in a program that is effective, safe, and meets your individual needs. You can also use these questions as a guide when selecting an exercise record or video cassette.

Do you recommend that I check with my doctor before I participate?

The answer should be more than Yes. In Aerobic Dancing, we've always encouraged and educated our students to follow these physical examination guidelines:

Under 30: If you're healthy and have had a complete checkup in the last year, then you can start exercising aerobically if you follow a program that promotes a safe, gradual progression.

30–39: Your physical examination should include a resting electrocardiogram made within three months of beginning an aerobic program.

40–50: Your physical examination, again within three months before starting an aerobic program, should include a resting *and* exercising electrocardiogram.

Over 50: You should check with your doctor immediately preceding your entering an aerobic program and he or she will advise you if you need to update your electrocardiogram tests.

We go a step further with prospective students by providing additional counseling for safe participation. For example, for those who are obviously overweight, we re-emphasize the importance of checking with their doctors, and advise them to participate at a walking level until their weight is within a healthy range.

Who develops or choreographs the program and what are his or her credentials?

The spokesperson should be happy and proud to give you a *specific* answer to this question. Remember, you're looking for a program designed by a professional.

How are your instructors trained?

Again, the answer should be straightforward and specific. My instructors must complete at least 80 hours of comprehensive training before they are certified to teach classes. They also must continually meet the following strict criteria. Each instructor must:

- be a non-smoker.
- maintain an optimal body weight.
- regularly pass a 12-minute running test in the "good" category.
- pass cardiopulmonary resuscitation training.

I'm a firm believer that fitness instructors should be positive examples of good health, because this helps motivate their students.

What is the class format?

If you're researching a program that labels itself "aerobic," it's important to know how much aerobic action is included in each class. An aerobic class should always include:

- 5–10 minutes to warm up,
- 20–30 minutes of continuous aerobic action, working large muscle groups,
- 5–10 minutes to cool down.

These are the components that enable a class to qualify as one of the four aerobic *workouts* you should have each week. If the aerobic action time (the time spent keeping your working heart rate in your desired range) is less than 20 minutes, then you're probably getting aerobic *benefits,* but not an aerobic *workout.* Let's use my Everyday Eights as an example. Completing the three segments will give you aerobic benefits. You expand this into an aerobic workout when you immediately go out for a walk or a run.

Is heart rate monitoring a part of the class format?

If the instructor does not ask students to periodically take their heart rates, then you cannot be assured that this is a safe and effective aerobic program.

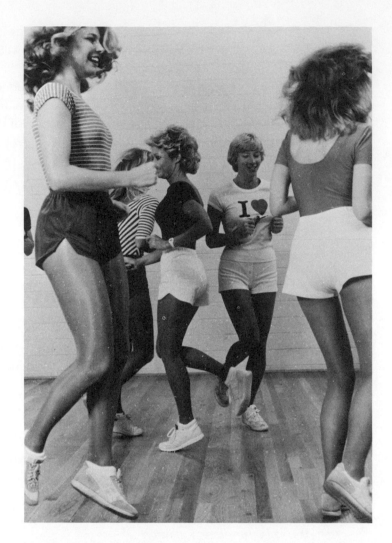

Also, it's not enough for instructors to simply ask students to time their heart rates. What counts is that the instructor monitor the results by observing students for signs of overexertion and by providing guidance on appropriate levels of participation.

May I observe a class?

This gives you the chance to see if the instructor is a professional. Does she or he provide the students with a good workout while being friendly, enthusiastic, motivating, and encouraging? Also, are the movements and patterns controlled, smoothly choreographed and enjoyable? Keep in mind that jerky movements and transitions can cause aches, pains, and even injuries.

Shop around until you discover your personal preferences. Then select a program that allows you to move not only aerobically but enjoyably, so you'll be motivated to stick with it. My students keep returning to one session after another because they see the results they're after—in their fitness and their figures—and because new music and new dances are introduced four times a year. It's this variety that keeps Aerobic Dancing challenging and exciting!

STEPPING UP YOUR PACE

Even though I'm trying to motivate you to acquire a more aerobic lifestyle, I certainly don't want to make you feel guilty if you're not currently involved in aerobic activities. The national passion for aerobics has given many people the notion that "If it's not aerobic, why spend your time on it?" My approach is you should feel good about *all* the things you do that are active, because not everything you do has to be aerobic. If you're a bowler, be happy that you're standing up and rolling the ball down the alley. If you love to play golf, feel wonderful that you're out walking in the fresh air and stretching your body when you swing. If you prefer to play social doubles in tennis, enjoy yourself! But don't count any of these sports as basic aerobic conditioners. Instead, look at them as positive things that you're doing for your body and your spirit. They add to your quality of life.

In a similar sense, if you're worried that lifting weights one day and doing yoga the next may not mix properly, my response would be: Why not do them both if you enjoy them? You're strengthening your muscles by lifting weights and you're working on flexibility with yoga, so that's a sensible combination. However, these two activities together will not provide a well-rounded *aerobic* program.

Of course, it may be that you're not involved in *any* type of physical activity outside your house or office. If so, here's a magic two-point program to get you going: first, learn my Everyday Eights and second, start walking! If you discover you can walk around the block only one time, don't be discouraged; you've made a start . . . now just try to add a minute a day, or a few extra yards, because every step counts!

Throughout this book I'm advocating a gentle approach to making changes in your lifestyle. Good and bad behavior patterns become habits over a period of time, and it takes *patience* to undo them or improve them. If you haven't exercised in five years, you can't expect to shape up in five days. And don't be intimidated by the challenge of getting into shape. Instead, take the attitude that *any* improvement is a step in the right direction. Eventually these steps add up, and you'll find that aerobic fitness can be as simple as a long walk three or four days a week.

The key here is not only to take that first step, but to strive for a slow, steady transition away from your sedentary habits. By implementing changes gradually, at your own pace, and avoiding the crash-diet approach to getting fit, you'll acquire a lifestyle change that is enduring.

EVERYDAY ENERGIZERS

If you're consciously trying to keep your weight under control, or making a concerted effort to lose weight, I *should* advise you to stop thinking about food and begin thinking about ways to move your body. But I can't do that. I love food and I can't put it out of my mind! Yet I do accept that I must DO certain things to get to the food. In fact, if you enjoy food and are reluctant to cut back or to moderate your eating, then why not increase your activity level sufficiently so you can still enjoy food *and* maintain a healthy, fit body. When you program more physical activity into your daily life, you not only feel better, you give yourself more eating opportunities.

I know that I use food as an incentive. I have even built an imaginary door in front of my eating opportunities and I have to do a certain amount of activity before I can go through that door. It's a game I play with myself . . . I get 200 calories if I pass GO. Thirty minutes of walking, which burns about 200 calories, is an eating opportunity that I can enjoy. So ask yourself: Are you keeping a balance between your energy input and your energy output? Or are you off balance? Are you going straight for the eating opportunities without doing the activities that open the door?

All my fitness career I've been interested in aerobic activity that benefits the heart, because that's the most important muscle in our bodies. But in this modern convenience-oriented world, we also need to think of ways to get more physical activity into our daily lives. I'm not saying you should chop wood, hang all your washing on a clothesline, or walk six miles to work. Instead, here are some Everyday Energizers, small, practical things that will make you feel better and allow you to have the fun of eating more food.

1. Try not to sit down when you're on the phone. I work at home and I stand or walk as I talk. I do this subconsciously now, but I had to think about it at first. Several years ago I read an article about Bob Hope, and when he was asked how he kept fit and young he said, "I tap-dance while I'm on the phone. I've done it for twenty years." That made me wonder, Why am I sitting down when I'm on the phone?—I'm a dancer, Bob Hope is a comedian; but he's tap-dancing while he's on the phone and I'm just trying to be funny.

2. I take the stairs at every opportunity. Neil and I live in a split-level house, and when we first moved in, I realized another exercise machine had entered my life—stairs. Yet in the beginning I would put everything in piles at each level, waiting until I HAD to go upstairs or downstairs. Since stair-climbing will actually burn about 10 to 20 calories a minute, I finally realized that instead of avoiding them I should take a positive approach and use them as a way to literally step *up* my life! Now I actually look for excuses to use them.

Try to take this same attitude toward stairs whenever you encounter them —in your home, when you're out shopping, or at work. (Are you in the habit of automatically taking the elevator or escalator just to go one or two floors?)

3. Add action breaks at work:
   —Stand up and pace or dance while on the telephone.
   —Have walking business meetings when the weather permits.
   —Go see coworkers face to face. This gets you up, and it's a friendlier

and more open way of communicating than over the phone or with a memo.

—At lunch, or on a coffee break, walk around the block or walk up the block and back, or walk across the street.

4. Before automatically getting in your car to run errands, ask yourself: "Is this something I could do on foot or by bicycle?" Then if you decide to drive, try parking a little farther away then usual and walking those extra steps— they will begin to add up.

5. For one week, when you're sitting down, try *not* to say those three little words, "While you're up ..." Instead, get up yourself and get what you need and perhaps even get something for someone else who says, "While you're up ..."

6. If you're with your spouse, kids, mom, dad, or a friend, waiting in a long line to see a popular movie, take turns walking around the block. (Just don't pick up an ice cream cone on your walk!)

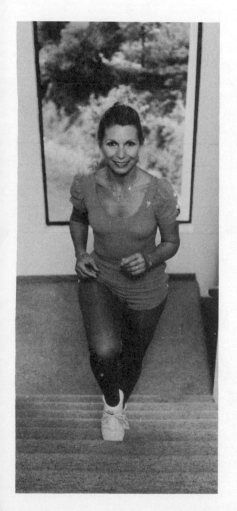

7. If you enjoy going to the beach, don't lie on the sand all the time. Even if you don't swim, you can still wade or take a walk and you'll also get the *top* of your shoulders suntanned.

8. Do you like to fish? I do! When I'm at my dad's in Florida I walk to the lake, put a minnow on my hook, take a brisk walk for about five minutes, then come back and check my bait. I call it Fitness Fishing! This also helps lessen my frustration when the fish keep "debating" my hook.

9. You've likely read a lot lately about the mental and physical benefits that a back-yard garden can yield: burning calories as you work out in the sun and fresh air, bending and stretching and digging away as you nurture your crop of fresh vegetables or flowers. This has always been my attitude, but a friend reminded me that gardening can also bring stress to one's life when treasured crops are afflicted by pests, runaway weeds, bad weather, or neighborhood kids caught up in a game of hide-and-seek. Keep that in mind if you've never had a chance to grow a garden. But if you have a green thumb, gopher it!

10. Look for ways to step up your pace on a seasonal basis. If it's spring and your child says, "Can we go out and fly my new kite?" that's something that will get your body moving in an unplanned way. Other play ideas? Well, there's Ping-Pong ... pool ... badminton ... croquet ... volleyball ... hopscotch ... swinging in the playground ... throwing a Frisbee ... doing somersaults down a grassy hill. Whatever you choose to do, this is recreation and relaxation, so don't worry about its being vigorous enough to be aerobic— just play!

11. In winter, try taking brisk walks in shopping malls. You'll avoid harsh weather and be entertained by people-watching and window shopping. (The same goes for hot summer days when you're not particularly keen on going outside for exercise.)

12. Another way to be more active during the "inside" days of winter is to do your spring cleaning in January. Then when spring bursts forth you'll have more time for *outside* action breaks.

13. When you're cleaning house, put on fast, peppy music that encourages you to work briskly. This is good for your body and you'll finish quicker. Try to take the same approach when doing yard work, washing the car, or sweeping the sidewalk.

14. Try "action cooking"! In sort of a joking way, I've suggested to my Aerobic Dancing students that they ought to put some favorite music on as they prepare dinner and perform some basic Aerobic Dancing steps, to "make your time in the kitchen more fun and get more exercise in the bargain." Now I find that some of my instructors are actually playing their session tapes and practicing dances while they cook.

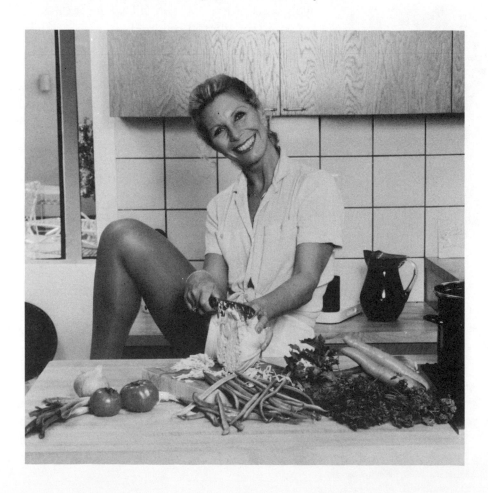

The whole point of "action cooking" is to move more instead of just standing around. It's easy: just swing your hips from side to side, do half–knee bends, one-steps or knee lifts. Cooking this way can also relieve stress, since chances are good you'll soon be laughing at yourself and that's a sure way to relax a little because now you're not taking yourself so seriously!

15. Are you an inefficient cook—like me? If so, don't feel guilty, just take heart at the fact that your inefficiency is burning extra calories. I love to cook, but for some reason I just can't seem to get it all together in the kitchen. I use twice as many pots and pans and bowls as I need to, and I take three times as many steps. I have no pattern that I follow from one meal to the next and I probably never will, yet I *welcome* this inefficiency because it keeps me more active and it's more spontaneous. Each big meal I prepare is an invigorating adventure. Who cares if it takes more energy? Who cares if all the dishes are dirty? I have an energy-saving device for this—called Neil.

16. When watching a television show, use breaks, slow spots, or commercials as a time to get up and exercise or at least be active. Here are a few ideas:

> —Reorganize a drawer.
> —Wash out a piece of clothing.
> —Do needlework.
> —Also, if you're a sports fan, jump, shout, or stand up and cheer when your team scores or makes a great play. Pretend you're at the game!

4

Aerobic Dancing Figure Eights

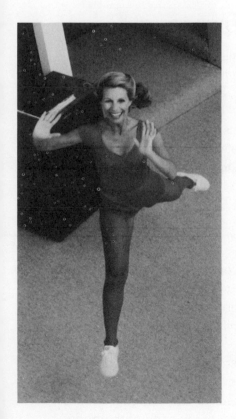

Aerobic Dancing is simple, vigorous dancing that gives you all the benefits of jogging plus figure-toning exercise. This chapter will give you a chance to sample the fun-filled flavor of my program by teaching you eight patterns I've choreographed for home use, drawing upon popular steps used in my classes.

I call these patterns "Figure Eights" because (1) you count the movements in eights, (2) the movements firm up your figure, (3) there are eight patterns; and (4) you'll be learning these patterns from eight of my instructors. These patterns are choreographed to capture the essence of a particular style and to match the mood of the suggested music.

Here are some ways to get the most out of the Figure Eights.

Do the first two segments of my Everyday Eights (the ten minutes of warm-up and floor work), then substitute these dance patterns for the last five-minute segment. Put on the suggested music for a specific pattern and dance the pattern once or twice. Then jog or walk around the room to pace yourself before dancing the pattern once or twice again. Continue following this system of dance-walk/jog until the music ends. Using two or three patterns in this way will give you an exhilarating and danceable ending to your Everyday Eights.

A second way to use these patterns is to go through the complete Everyday Eights and then expand them to an aerobic workout of 20 to 30 minutes by using the same system of dance-walk/jog. This is a no-excuses alternative when you can't go *outdoors* to continue exercising.

Third, you may want to repeat certain patterns more than others to emphasize *specific* figure-firming features. In this way you can individualize your exercise session and tackle particular areas of your body. Even though these Aerobic Dancing Figure Eights involve as many parts of the body as possible, some patterns spotlight certain areas. For example, you may want to concentrate on really stretching your upper body when doing the "Stretch 'n' Reach" pattern, and to concentrate on working your lower body when you "Polka." By choosing the patterns and the number of repetitions that meet *your* needs, it's easy to customize the Figure Eights.

Fourth, if you've been dancing up a storm with my first book, you can now expand your Aerobic Dancing repertoire by adding these new steps and styles. This can give you a new challenge—and variety.

Fifth, you can string all the patterns together, do each one twice, and end up with an aerobic segment that lasts five to six minutes. This won't be a choreographed dance, but all the different styles and moods will make you feel like part of a vaudeville show!

Sixth, as with all my Aerobic Dancing programs, it's important to remember that you can do these patterns at a walking level by simply eliminating the hopping, jumping and bouncing action. This will still give you a good workout for both figure and fitness.

WHY AEROBIC DANCING IS SO POPULAR

At age five, although I was already an avid little dancer, I wasn't dreaming about creating Aerobic Dancing. But I had other dreams that paved the way to what I've done. By the time I was twenty-five, I was sick of hearing people say, "I can't dance," "I hate to exercise," and "I don't have time to stay in shape." So I was determined to create a fitness program that would make people jump with joy. And now I have students everywhere saying, "I can dance! . . . Fitness can be fun! . . . I look forward to every class! . . . I'm *finding* the time to stay in shape!"

There are a number of reasons why Aerobic Dancing appeals to so many people and why they just keep on dancin':

—My specialty is choreographing dances for non-dancers. So, skill and technique are not important; you do everything at your own level of ability and at your own level of aerobic effort: the walking level, the jogging level, or the running level. If you can clap, walk, and lift your knees, you can get through an Aerobic Dance.

—I emphasize play, not perfection, but I also realize there's a wonderful feeling of success that comes after learning a new pattern.

—I know you don't want your time wasted, so my unique get-it-all-together concept saves you time by exercising as many parts of the body at once as possible.

—The arms usually get very little exercise when you jog or walk, but in Aerobic Dancing choreographed arm movements add upper-body toning.

—Remember, when you're dancing you burn more calories than you would by spending the same amount of time exercising on the floor.

—I make shaping up and keeping in shape an exhilarating experience because you're not simply exercising to music; you're actually dancing choreographed dances that make you feel as if you're part of the music.

—Many times we've had three generations from one family taking Aerobic Dancing at the same time (grandmother, mother, and daughter)—which proves that you can do this at any age, at your own level.

I've always felt that the heart of Aerobic Dancing is FUN, since that's what makes you stick with it week after week, year after year. Maintaining figure firmness and fitness is a lifetime opportunity, so what good is the most effective program if you get bored with it, treat it as a chore, and finally get burned out and quit?

So join the fun and learn the Figure Eights!

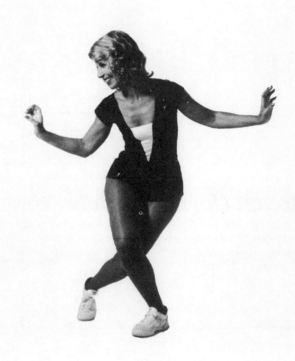

STRETCH 'N' REACH PATTERN

LEARN THESE STEPS:

Stretch Up, Cross Over

(directions for facing front and moving to the right)

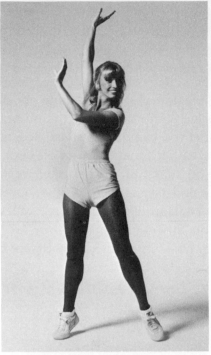 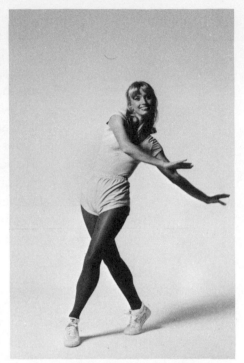

Count: 1 — Begin with feet together, weight on left foot, hands close in front of chest. Step up on **right** foot to right side as arms circle counterclockwise up to overhead.

2 — Draw **left** foot in front of right as knees bend a bit and arms continue circling around and down to left side.

Stretch Up, Cross Over

(directions for facing front and moving to the left)

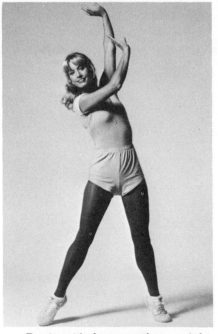 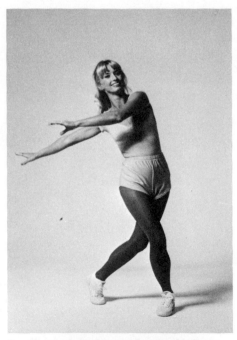

1 — Begin with feet together, weight on right foot, hands close in front of chest. Step up on **left** foot to left side as arms circle clockwise up to overhead.

2 — Draw **right** foot in front of left as knees bend a bit and arms continue circling around and down to right side.

Shoulder Rolls, Single

(directions for right and left)

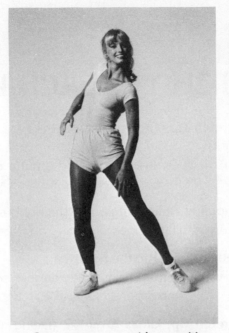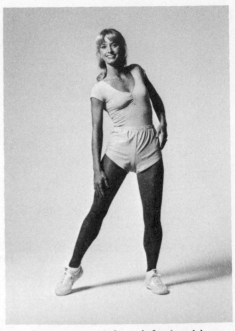

Step out to stride position, hands resting on front of thighs.
1 Body sways **right** as right shoulder rolls up, back, down and around in a continuous motion.

2 Body sways **left** as left shoulder rolls up, back, down and around in a continuous motion.

Reach Big

(directions for right and for left)

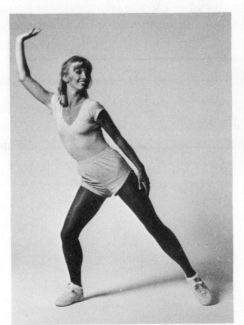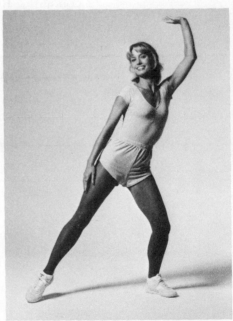

Begin with feet in stride position, arms down at sides relaxed.
1 Stretch right arm up, around and down *clockwise* as body
2 sways **right** and right knee bends a bit.

1 Stretch left arm up, around and down *counterclockwise* as
2 body sways **left** and left knee bends a bit.

(continued)

STRETCH 'N' REACH PATTERN

(4 counts)   **Stretch Up, Cross Over—2** (facing front and moving to the right)
        Arms: Circle arms up and around *counterclockwise* once for each Stretch Up, Cross Over.

(2 counts)   **Shoulder Rolls, Single—to the right, to the left**
        Arms: Hands loosely resting on front of thighs

(2 counts)   **Reach Big—1** to the right
        Arms: Left arm down at side relaxed; right arm reaches up and around *clockwise.*

(4 counts)   **Stretch Up, Cross Over—2** (facing front and moving to the left)
        Arms: Circle arms up and around *clockwise* once for each Stretch Up, Cross Over.

(2 counts)   **Shoulder Rolls, Single—to the left, to the right**
        Arms: Hands resting loosely on front of thighs

(2 counts)   **Reach Big—1** to the left
        Arms: Right arm down at side relaxed; left arm reaches up and around *counterclockwise.*

Suggested Music: "Key Largo" by Bertie Higgins, from *Just Another Day in Paradise.*

Body Benefits: Shapes up arms, waist, hips, legs, inner and outer thighs. Aerobic benefits from stretching and steppin' out!

Instructor: Rochelle Munson

50s PATTERN

LEARN THESE STEPS:

Two-Step "Stroll-It"

(directions for right)

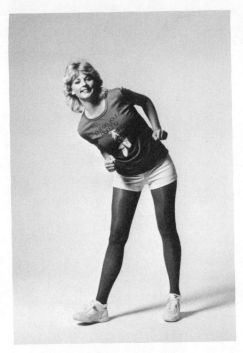

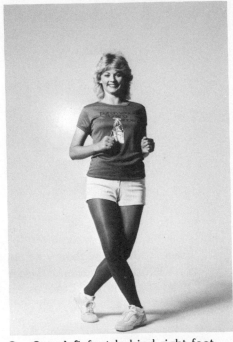

Count: 1 Begin with feet together, weight on left foot, arms in "ready-to-jog" position. Step **right** foot to right side with a rolling heel-toe motion, keeping right leg straight and leaning right a bit.

2 Step **left** foot behind right foot, bending both knees.

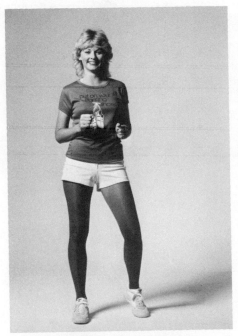

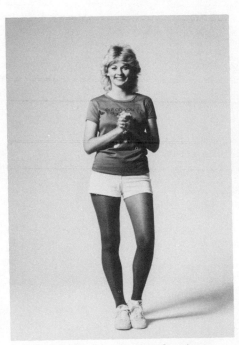

3 Step **right** foot to right side.

4 Pull **left** foot in to right foot keeping weight on right foot and clap hands close in front of chest.

(Reverse to do moving left.)

(continued)

Jog "Wild"

(directions for two)

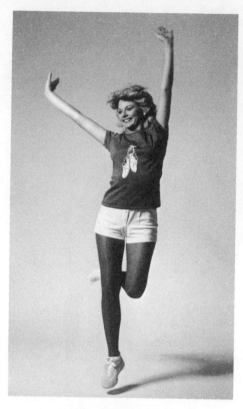

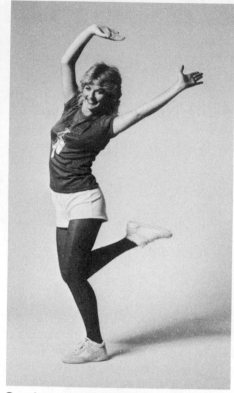

1 Begin with feet together, weight on left foot, arms extended overhead. Jog onto **right** foot as extended arms sway to right side vigorously.

2 Jog onto **left** foot as extended arms sway to left side vigorously.

Kick "Cool"

(directions for two)

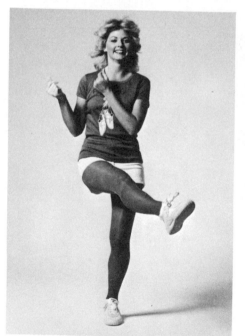

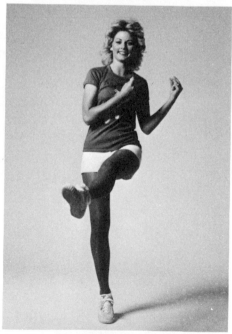

1 Begin with feet together, weight on left foot, hands close in front of chest. Hop on **left** foot as you kick right foot forward LOW and hands swing up to right shoulder and fingers snap. Jump to **right** foot, as left foot prepares to kick.

1 Hop on **right** foot as you kick left foot forward LOW and hands swing up to left shoulder and fingers snap. Jump to **left** foot, as right foot prepares to kick.

50s PATTERN

(16 counts)   **Two-Step "Stroll-It"—to the right, to the left, to the right, to the left** (4 counts each)
     Arms: Close ready-to-jog position; clap on each 4th count.

(8 counts)   **Jog "Wild"—8** turning in a full circle right
     Arms: Extended overhead, arms sway side to side vigorously.

(8 counts)   **Kick "Cool"—4** (2 counts each)
     Arms: Swing hands from shoulder to shoulder; right, left, right, left; end each swing with a finger-snap.

Suggested music: "Back to School Again" by The Four Tops, from *Grease II.*

Body benefits: Shapes up arms, waist, hips, seat, legs, fronts of thighs, backs of thighs, inner and outer thighs. Aerobic benefits from jogging, hopping, jumping and steppin' out!

Instructor: Carey Skinner

DISCO CHARLESTON PATTERN

LEARN THESE STEPS:

Disco Charleston

(directions for one)

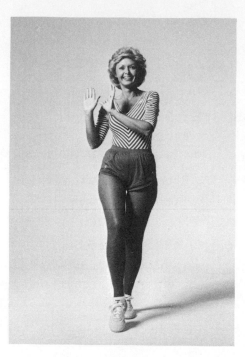

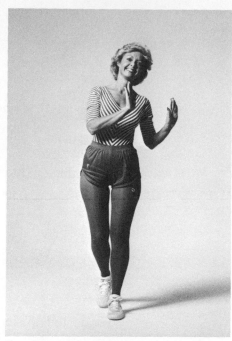

Count: Begin with feet together, weight on left foot, hands close in front of chest, palms facing out.

1 Touch **right** foot forward as arms swing to the right.

2 Step **right** foot back as arms swing to the left.

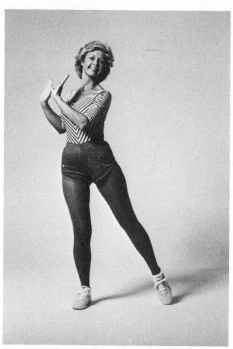

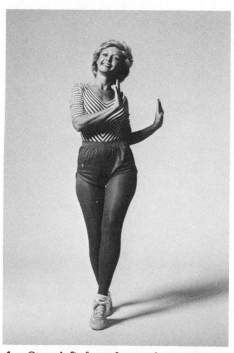

3 Touch **left** foot *out to left side* as arms swing to the right.

4 Step **left** foot forward as arms swing to the left.

Break Slow

(directions for one)

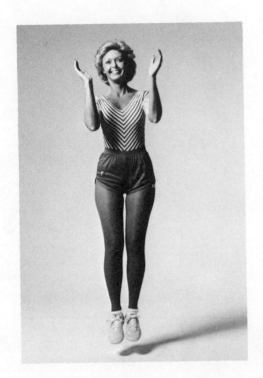

1 Jump up, keeping feet together. As feet **land,** clap hands close in front of chest, keeping knees re-

and laxed, then add a small **bounce.**

(continued)

Disco Swing

(directions for two)

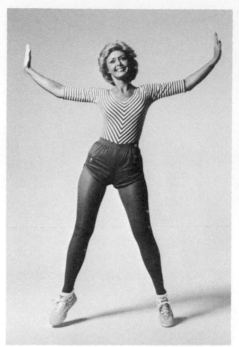 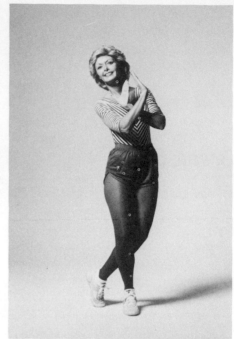

1   Begin with feet together, weight on left foot, hands close in front of chest. Step **right** foot wide to right side as arms swing out at sides to head level, palms out.

2   Touch **left** foot *behind* right foot as arms swing down and cross close in front of chest, palms out.

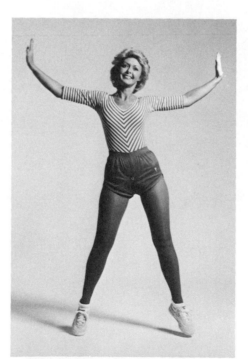 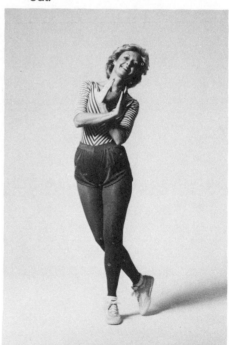

1   Step **left** foot wide to left side as arms swing out at sides to head level, palms out.

2   Touch **right** foot *behind* left foot as arms swing down and cross close in front of chest, palms out. TO ADD SOME BOUNCE: Each time you Touch and each time you Step do it with a bouncy, lively feeling.

DISCO CHARLESTON PATTERN

(12 counts)   **Disco Charleston—3** (4 counts each)
           Arms: Swing both arms side to side, close to body.

(4 counts)   **Break Slow—4,** turning in place in a full circle right (1 count each)
           Arms: Clap once for each Break.

(12 counts)   **Disco Swing—6** (2 counts each)
           Arms: Swing arms out at sides to head level, then swing down to cross close in front of chest for each Disco Swing.

(4 counts)   **Break Slow—4,** turning in place in a full circle right (1 count each)
           Arms: Clap once for each Break.

Suggested music: "Break Down the Door" by Barry Manilow, from *I Should Love You Again.*

Body benefits: Shapes up arms, legs, inner and outer thighs. Aerobic benefits from jumping, bouncing and steppin' out!

Instructor: Sally Levy

PAC-MAN PATTERN

LEARN THESE STEPS:

Hustle Jog

(directions for one forward and backward set)

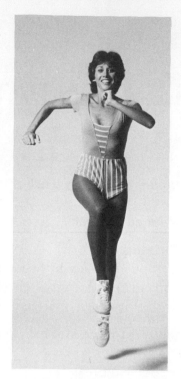
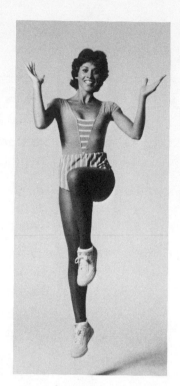

Begin with feet together, weight on left foot, arms in ready-to-jog position. Jog 3 steps forward, **right-left-right.**

Count:

1,2,3

4 Hop on **right** foot as you lift left knee and clap hands close in front of chest.

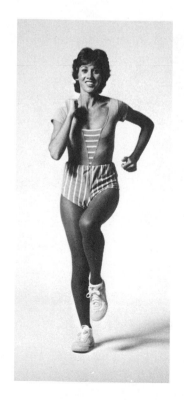
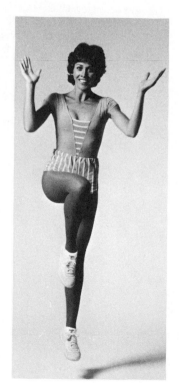

5,6 Jog 3 steps backward, **left-right-**
7 **left.**

8 Hop on **left** foot as you lift right knee and clap hands close in front of chest.

Jog "Play It"

(directions for 8, turning in a full circle right)

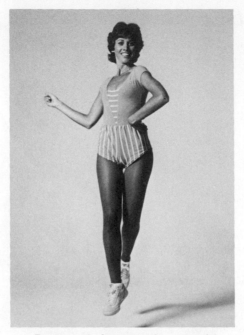

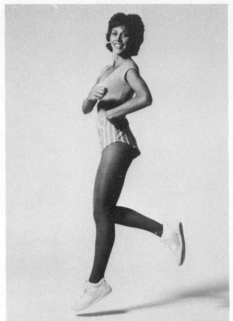

1 Begin with feet together, weight on left foot, left hand on hip, right arm in ready-to-jog position. Get ready to jog 8 steps in a full circle right. Jog **right** as right arm swings out to right side, keeping elbow close.

2 Jog **left** as right arm swings across, ending in front of body with elbow close. This is how you "play" side to side. Repeat

3,4 jogging **right** and **left** with side-to-side arms so you've completed 4 jogs in a half circle right.

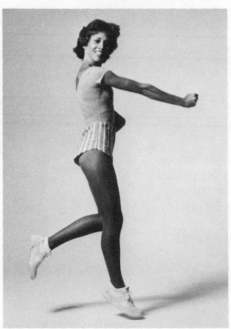

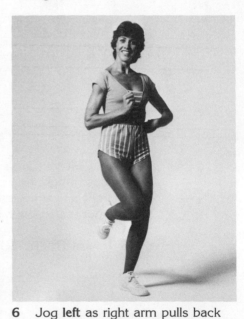

5 Jog **right** as right arm extends forward.

6 Jog **left** as right arm pulls back in. This is how you "play" forward and backward. Repeat jog-

7,8 ging **right** and **left** with forward and backward arms so you've completed a total of 8 jogs and you've finished a full circle right.

(continued)

Four-Step "Eat the Dots"

(directions for right)

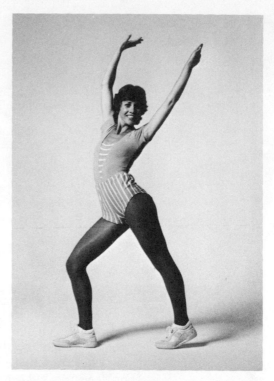

1   Begin with feet together, weight on left foot, hands close in front of chest. Step **right** foot wide to right side (toes pointing right as toes of left foot swivel to face right and arms swing out at sides and extend overhead with elbows relaxed.

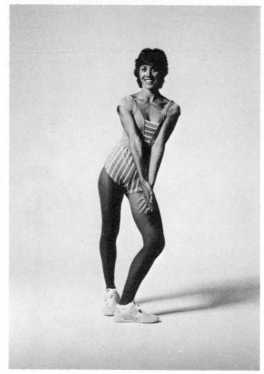

2   Pull **left** foot in to right foot as toes of right foot swivel to face front and arms swing down at sides to clap low in front of body.

3,4
5,6   Repeat THREE MORE TIMES.
7,8

(Reverse to do moving left.)

PAC-MAN PATTERN

(8 counts)   **Hustle Jog—1** forward and backward set
               Arms: Ready-to-jog position; clap on each hop.

(8 counts)   **Jog "Play-It"—8** turning in a full circle right
               Arms: Left hand on hip; right hand "plays" side to side 2
               times; then right arm "plays" forward and backward
               2 times.

(16 counts)   **Four-Step "Eat The Dots"—to the right, to the left** (8 counts
               each)
               Arms: Swing arms up to overhead, then swing down to end
               with a clap low in front of body 4 times for each Four-
               Step set.

Suggested music: "Pac-Man Fever" by Buckner and Garcia, from *Pac-Man
Fever.*

Body benefits: Shapes up arms, waist, hips, seat, legs, fronts of thighs, backs
of thighs, inner and outer thighs. Aerobic benefits from jogging, hopping and steppin' out!

Instructor: Janci Farwell

POLKA PATTERN

LEARN THESE STEPS:

Polka Combo

(directions for right)

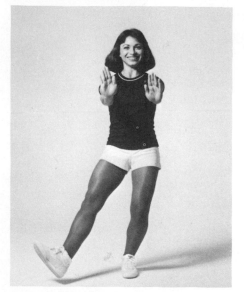 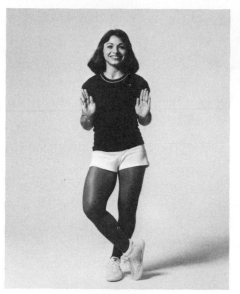 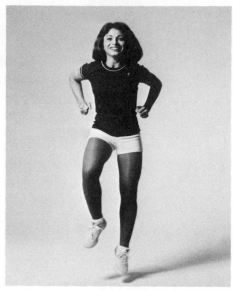

Count:
1 Begin with feet together, arms in ready-to-jog position. Hop on **left** foot as you touch right heel to right diagonal and arms push forward.

2 Hop on **left** foot as you touch-point right toe in front of left foot and arms pull in.
3,4 Repeat these 2 hops.

and
5 With arms in ready-to-jog position, hop on **left** foot as you lift right knee a bit, then step **right** foot to right side.

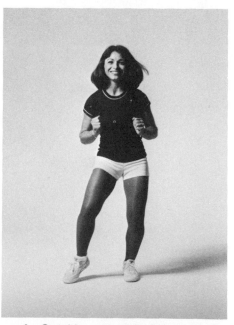 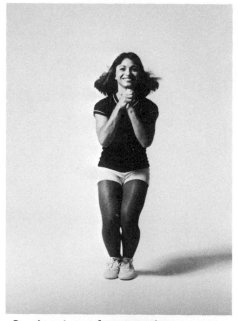

and
6
and 7 Quickly step **left** foot next to right foot with a small jump and step **right** foot to right side. Repeat once again,

8 then jump feet **together.** (Reverse directions to move left.)

Jump/Half-Turn

(directions for one to end facing the rear)

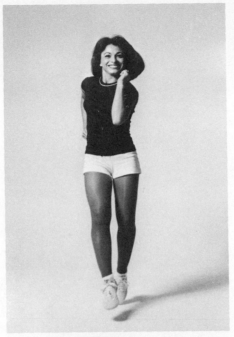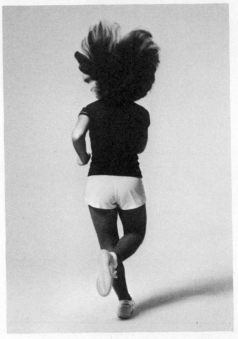

1   Begin with feet together, weight on left foot, arms in ready-to-jog position. Jump forward onto **right** foot, keeping left foot close to the ground.

2   Pivot body in a half-turn left to face rear and jump onto **left** foot.

Break Fast

(directions for one)

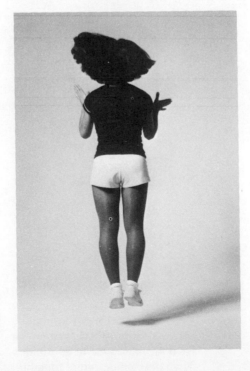

1   Jump up, keeping feet together. As feet **land,** clap hands close in front of chest, keeping knees relaxed.

(continued)

Jump/Half-Turn

(directions for one to end facing the front)

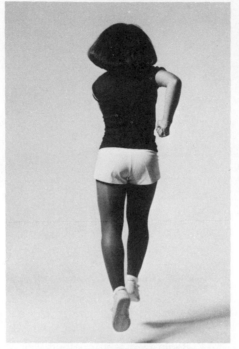
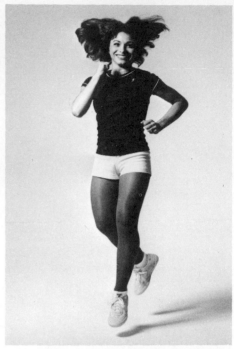

1 Begin with feet together, weight on left foot, arms in ready-to-jog position. Jump forward onto **right** foot, keeping left foot close to the ground.

2 Pivot body in a half-turn left to face front and jump onto **left** foot.

Knee-Lift Hopping

(directions for two)

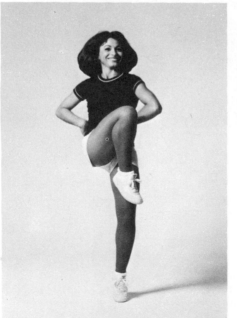
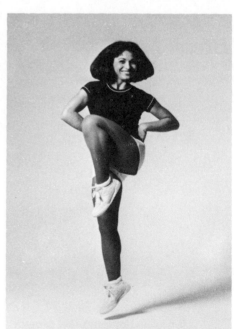

1 Begin with feet together, hands on hips. Hop on **left** foot as you lift right knee and left shoulder.
2 Then bounce **both feet** together.

1 Hop on **right** foot as you lift left knee and right shoulder. Then
2 bounce **both feet** together.

POLKA PATTERN

(16 counts)   **Polka Combo—to the right, to the left** (8 counts each)
           Arms: Push-pull arms on each heel-toe, then hold arms in
           ready-to-jog position.

(2 counts)   **Jump/Half-Turn—1** (to end facing the *rear*)
           Arms: Ready-to-jog position

(2 counts)   **Break Fast—2** (facing the *rear*) (one count each)
           Arms: Clap once for each Break.

(2 counts)   **Jump/Half-Turn—1** (to end facing the *front*)
           Arms: Ready-to-jog position

(2 counts)   **Break Fast—2** (facing the *front*)
           Arms: Clap once for each Break.

(8 counts)   **Knee-Lifts Hopping—4** (2 counts each)
           Arms: Hands on hips with alternating shoulder lifts

Suggested music: "America" by Neil Diamond, from *Jazz Singer.*

Body benefits: Shapes up arms, legs, seat, front of thighs, back of thighs, inner and outer thighs. Aerobic benefits from hopping, jumping and bouncing.

Instructor: Sylvia Althaus

THERE'S NO STOPPING YOU! PATTERN

LEARN THESE STEPS:

Thigh Rock Double "Stop-Hand"

(directions for three)

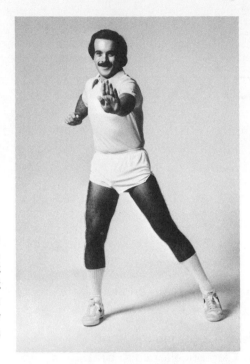

Count:

Begin with feet in stride position, hands close in front of chest, palms front. Energetically shift

1 weight to **right** foot, keeping left foot on the floor as left arm pushes forward and right elbow

2 pulls back. **Bounce** once in this position.

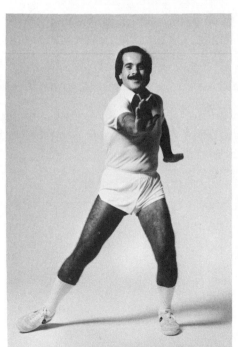

1 Energetically shift weight to **left** foot, keeping right foot on the floor as right arm pushes forward and left arm pulls in with

2 elbow back. **Bounce** once in this position.

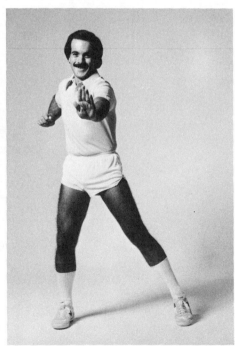

1 Energetically shift weight to **right** foot, keeping left foot on the floor as left arm pushes forward and right arm pulls in with

2 elbow back. **Bounce** once in this position.

Break Fast

(directions for one)

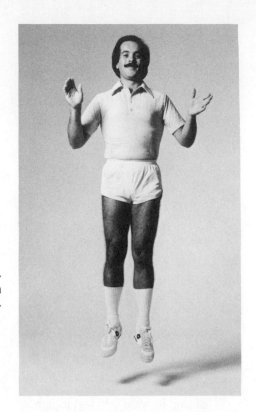

1   Jump up, keeping feet together. As feet **land,** clap hands close in front of chest, keeping knees relaxed.

Slide

(directions for one set of 4 to the right)

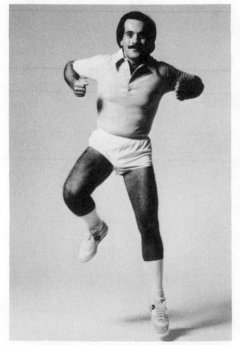 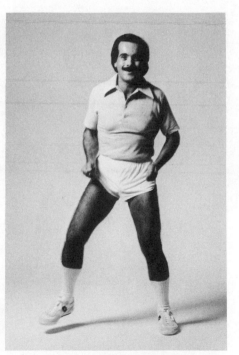 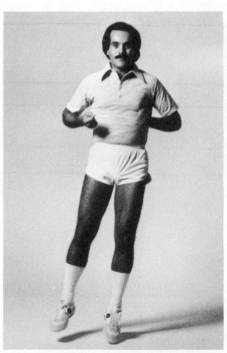

and Begin with feet together, arms in ready-to-jog position. Hop on **left** foot as you lift right knee a bit,

1   then step **right** foot to right side.

and Quickly bring **left** foot next to right foot with a small jump and
2   step **right** foot to right side.
and 3 Repeat this two more times.
and 4

(Reverse to do moving left.)

(continued)

Jump Forward,
Jump Back

(directions for one)

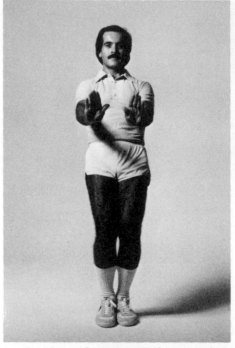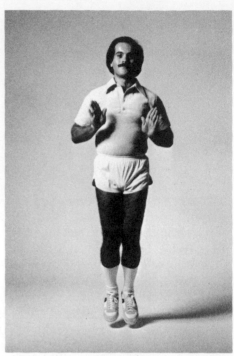

1 Jump **forward** with feet together, knees slightly flexed as arms push forward.

2 Jump **back** with feet together, knees slightly flexed as arms pull in.

Jumping Jack

(directions for one)

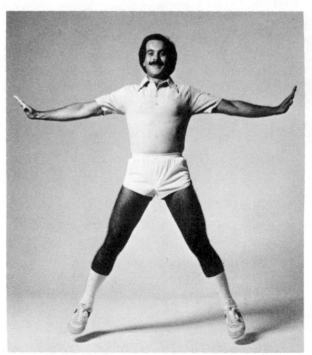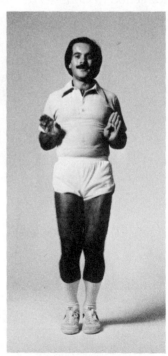

Begin with feet together, hands close in front of chest. Jump
1 lightly to **stride** position as arms push out at sides.

2 Jump feet **together** as arms pull in.

THERE'S NO STOPPING YOU!
PATTERN

(6 counts) **Thigh Rock Double—3** (2 counts each)
               Arms: "Stop-Hand"—left single push forward for 2 counts, right forward for 2 counts, then left forward for 2 counts.

(2 counts) **Break Fast—2** (one count each)
               Arms: Clap hands once for each Break.

(6 counts) **Thigh Rock Double—3**
               Arms: "Stop-Hand"—left single push forward for 2 counts, right forward for 2 counts, then left forward for 2 counts.

(2 counts) **Break Fast—2**
               Arms: Clap hands once for each Break.

(4 counts) **Slides—1** set of 4, moving to the right
               Arms: Ready-to-jog position

(2 counts) **Jump Forward, Jump Back—1**
               Arms: Push forward and pull in.

(2 counts) **Jumping Jack—1**
               Arms: Push out at sides and pull in.

(4 counts) **Slides—1** set of 4, moving to the left
               Arms: Ready-to-jog position

(2 counts) **Jump Forward, Jump Back—1**
               Arms: Push forward and pull in.

(2 counts) **Jumping Jack—1**
               Arms: Push out at sides and pull in.

Suggested music: "There's No Stopping Us" by Sister Sledge, from *The Sisters*

Body benefits: Shapes up arms, hips, front of thighs, back of thighs, inner and outer thighs. Aerobic benefits from bouncing, sliding, jumping and hopping.

Instructor: John Lewis, Jr.

WORKOUT PATTERN

LEARN THESE STEPS:

Hustle Jog

(directions for one forward and backward set)

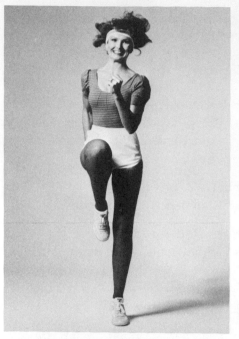

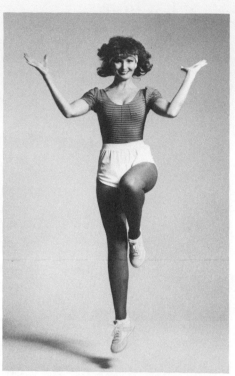

Count: 1 2,3 Begin with feet together, weight on left foot, arms in ready-to-jog position. Jog 3 forward, **right-left-right.**

4 Hop on **right** foot as you lift left knee and clap hands close in front of chest.

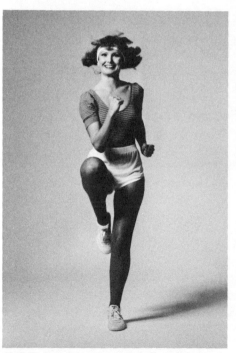

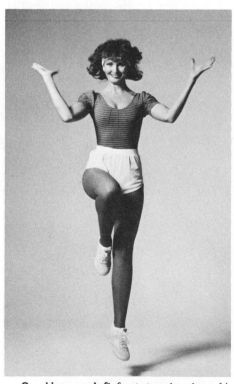

5,6,7 Jog 3 backward, **left-right-left.**

8 Hop on **left** foot, turning in a ¼ *circle right* as you lift right knee and clap hands close in front of chest.

Four-Step "Lift Two Weights"

(directions for right)

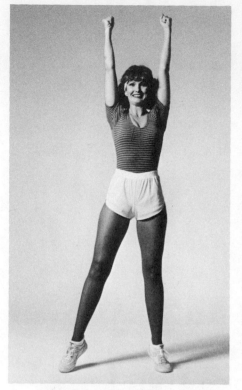

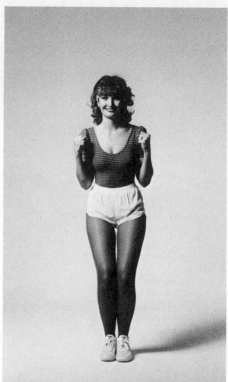

Begin with weight on left foot, fists close in front of shoulders.

1 Step **right** foot to right side as arms "lift weights" straight up to overhead.

2 Pull **left** foot in to right foot as arms pull weights down, close in
3,4 front of shoulders. Repeat step-
5,6 ping right-left THREE MORE
7,8 TIMES.

(Reverse to do moving left.)

Two-Step "Lift One Weight"

(directions for right)

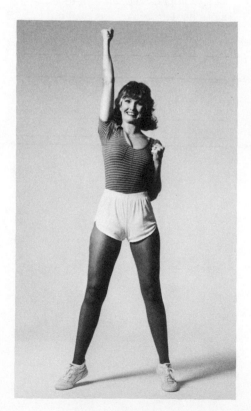

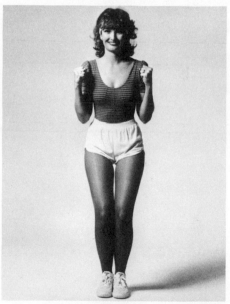

Begin with feet together, weight on left foot, fists close in front of
1 shoulders. Step **right** foot to right side as right arm "lifts weight" straight up to overhead.

2 Pull **left** foot in to right foot as right arm pulls weight down, close in front of shoulder. Re-
3 peat, stepping **right** foot to right side, lifting weight, and then
4 pulling **left** foot in to right foot, pulling weight down.

(continued)

Two-Step "Lift One Weight"

(directions for left)

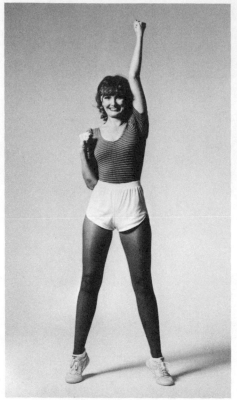 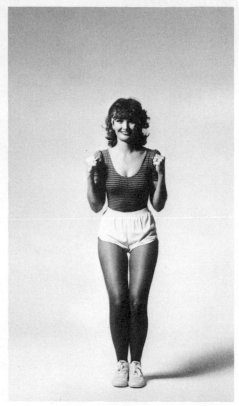

1 Begin with feet together, weight on right foot, fists close in front of shoulders. Step **left** foot to left side as left arm "lifts weight" straight up to overhead.

2 Pull **right** foot in to left foot as left arm pulls weight down, close in front of shoulders. Repeat
3 once, stepping **left** foot to left side, lifting weight, and then
4 pulling **right** foot in to left foot, pulling weight down.

WORKOUT PATTERN

(32 counts) **Hustle Jog—4** forward and backward sets (8 counts each)
Arms: Ready-to-jog position, clap on each hop. Make a square by turning ¼ turn right each time you hop on left foot.

(16 counts) **Four-Step "Lift Two Weights"—to the right, to the left** (8 counts each)
Arms: Fists shoot up and pull in 4 times each way.

(16 counts) **Two-Step "Lift One Weight"—to the right, to the left, to the right, to the left** (4 counts each)
Arms: Left arm in close ready-to-jog position; right fist shoots up and pulls in 2 times when moving right. Then right arm in close ready-to-jog position; left fist shoots up and pulls in 2 times when moving left.

Suggested music: "Be Your Own Hero" by the kids from *Fame, Fame* Soundtrack.

Body benefits: Shapes up arms, waist, hips, seat, legs, front of thighs, back of thighs, inner and outer thighs. Aerobic benefits from jogging, hopping and steppin' out!

Instructor: Kathy Miller

SWING-OUT PATTERN

LEARN THESE STEPS:

Cha-Cha "Swing-Out"

(directions for one)

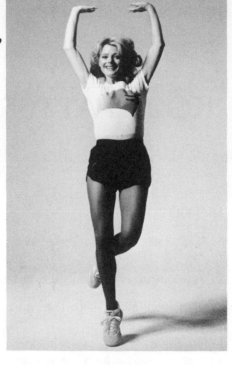

Count:
1
2

Begin with feet together, weight on left foot, hands close in front of chest. Step forward onto **right** foot as arms swing out at sides up to overhead. Step **left** foot in place.

3 and 4 Do 3 fast, low jogs in place, **right-left-right,** as arms swing down at sides and cross close in front of chest.

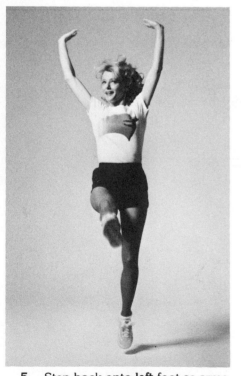

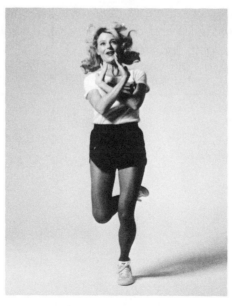

5
6

Step back onto **left** foot as arms swing out at sides up to overhead. Step **right** foot in place.

7 and 8 Do 3 fast, low jogs in place, **left-right-left,** as arms swing down at sides and cross close in front of chest. To add some bounce: Each time you "step" do it with a bouncy, lively feeling.

Jump/Half-Turn

(directions for two, to make a complete turn to the left)

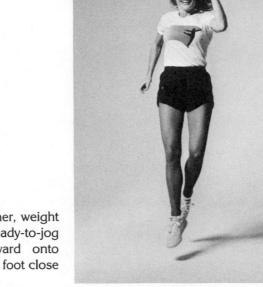

Begin with feet together, weight on left foot, arms in ready-to-jog position. Jump forward onto
1 **right** foot, keeping left foot close to the ground.

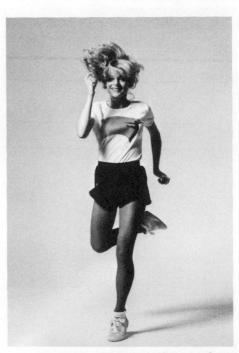

Pivot body in a half-turn left to
2 face rear and jump onto **left** foot.

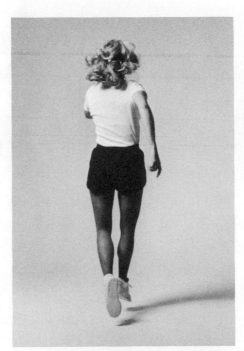

1 Jump forward onto **right** foot again, keeping left foot close to the ground.

Pivot body in a half-turn left to
2 face front and jump onto **left** foot.

(continued)

Break Slow

(directions for one)

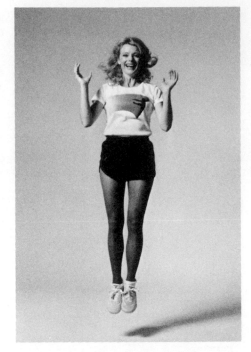

Jump up, keeping feet together.

1 As feet **land,** clap hands close in front of chest, keeping knees re-

2 laxed, then add a small **bounce.**

Slide 'n' Step Back "Swing-Out"

(directions for one)

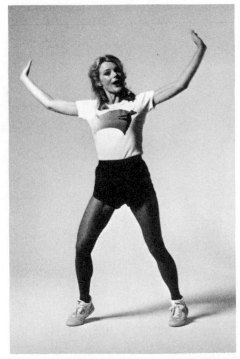

1 Begin with feet together, weight on left foot, hands close in front of chest. Step **right** foot to right side as arms begin to swing out at side.

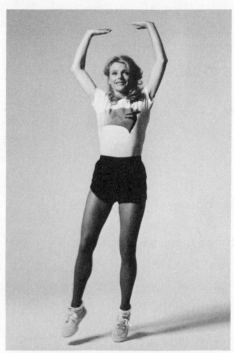

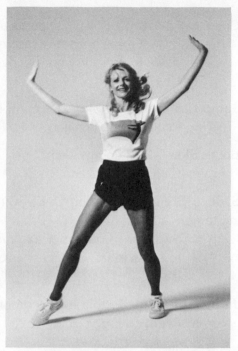

and Quick-jump **left** foot next to right foot as arms continue up to overhead, then

2 step **right** foot to right side as arms begin to swing down at sides.

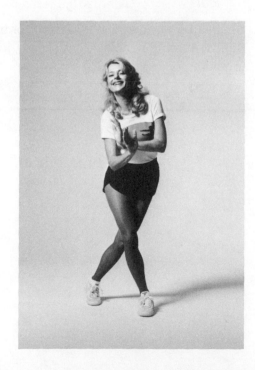

3 Step **left** foot *back behind* right
4 foot, then step **right** foot in place as arms continue swinging down at sides and cross close in front of chest.

(Reverse to do moving left.)

(continued)

139

SWING-OUT PATTERN

(24 counts)   **Cha-Cha "Swing-Out"—3** (8 counts each)
           Arms: Swing arms out at sides to overhead, then swing down to cross in front of chest 2 times for each Cha-Cha.

(4 counts)   **Jump/Half-Turn—2** (to make a complete turn to the left)
           Arms: Ready-to-jog position

(4 counts)   **Break Slow—2** (2 counts each)
           Arms: Clap once for each Break.

(24 counts)   **Slide 'n' Step Back "Swing-Out"—6** (4 counts each) alternating to right and left
           Arms: Swing arms out at sides to overhead then swing down to cross in front of chest once for each Slide 'n' Step Back.

(4 counts)   **Jump/Half-Turn—2** (to make a complete turn to the left)
           Arms: Ready-to-jog position

(4 counts)   **Break Slow—2**
           Arms: Clap once for each Break.

Suggested music: "Make a Move on Me" by Olivia Newton-John, from *Physical.*

Body benefits: Shapes up arms, waist, legs, front of thighs, inner and outer thighs. Aerobic benefits from sliding, jumping, bouncing and jogging.

Instructor: Kim Fitzgerald

5

A Chance to Dance!

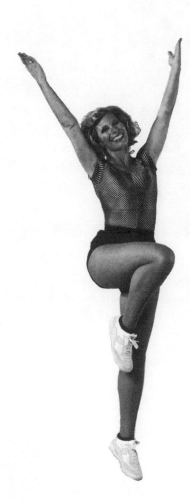

I have my chance to dance when I choreograph four new sessions each year. When I wake up in the morning and it's time to start working on the first dance, I think to myself, Wow!—this is my life—my chance to create, to share, to move in new ways, to experience new feelings. I suit up, leap in front of my studio mirrors, and shout, "THE CHOREOGRAPHER IS IN!"

If you're not already one of my students, here's your chance to really get into a "dance." And, if you're in my program, here's an entertaining way to add aerobic activity to your week. I've combined five patterns from Chapter Four with several new transition patterns that I'll teach you in this chapter. This dance gives you a great way to add aerobic action and figure toning to your fitness plan. Why not use it as a five-minute aerobic finale to your workout, whether it's the Everyday Eights, jogging, playing tennis, walking, skiing, cycling, or any aerobic activity you love?

No matter how you put this dance to use, the fun of letting yourself go, kicking up your heels, and pretending and playing will leave you on an emotional and physical high. I have choreographed this dance to cut one, side one, Part One, of "Hooked on Classics" (by Louis Clark conducting the Royal Philharmonic Orchestra, RCA). So use "Hooked on Classics" as an exercise treat and you'll get hooked on Aerobic Dancing!

Now put on your rehearsal outfit and get ready to learn a five-minute Aerobic Dance that's a real production!

First, I'll teach you the:

- **Introduction Pattern**
- **Pacing Pattern**
- **Rainbow Pattern**
- **Long Pacing Pattern**
- **Hi-Ho-Silver Pattern**
- **Hallelujah Pattern** and
- **Finale Pattern**

Next, a quick review of these patterns you just learned in Chapter Four:

- **50s Pattern**
- **Polka Pattern**
- **There's No Stopping You! Pattern**
- **Workout Pattern and**
- **Swing-Out Pattern**

All set? Let's begin!

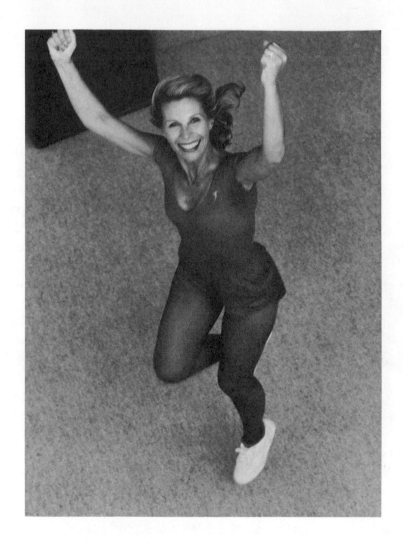

INTRODUCTION PATTERN

LEARN THESE STEPS:

Shoulder Rolls, Single

(directions for right and left)

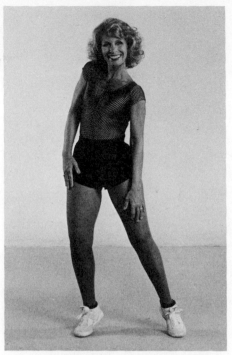 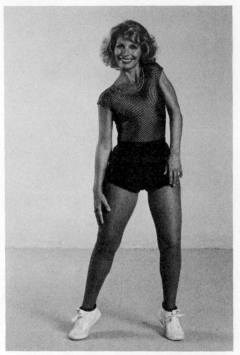

Count: 1   Begin with feet in stride position, hands loosely resting on front of thighs. As body sways **right,** right shoulder rolls up, back, down and around in a continuous motion.

2   As body sways **left,** left shoulder rolls up, back, down and around in a continuous motion.

Break Slow

(Directions for one)

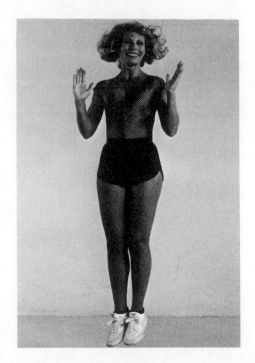

Jump up, keeping feet together.
1 As feet **land,** clap hands close in front of chest, keeping knees relaxed, then add a small **bounce.**
2

(continued)

Kick "Cool"

(directions for two)

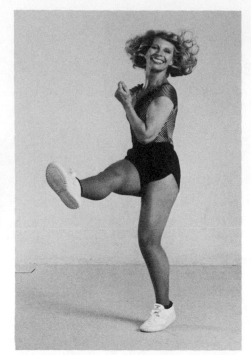

1   Begin with feet together, weight on left foot, hands close in front of chest. Hop on **left** foot as you kick right foot forward LOW and arms swing up to right shoulder and fingers snap. Jump to **right**
2   foot, as left foot prepares to kick.

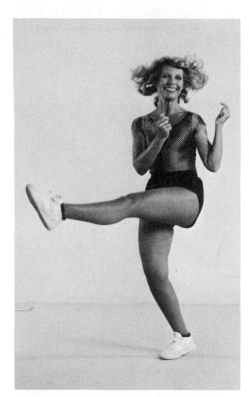

1   Hop on **right** foot as you kick left foot forward LOW and arms swing up to left shoulder and fin-
2   gers snap. Jump to **left** foot, as right foot prepares to kick.

INTRODUCTION PATTERN

Wait for the music—3 counts!

(2 counts)   **Shoulder Rolls, Single—right and left**
     Arms: Hands loosely resting on front of thighs

(3 counts)   Wait 3 counts!

(2 counts)   **Shoulder Rolls, Single—right and left**
     Arms: Hands loosely resting on front of thighs

(3 counts)   Wait 3 counts!

(6 counts)   **Shoulder Rolls, Single—6 alternating right and left**
     Arms: Hands loosely resting on front of thighs

(8 counts)   **Break Slow—4** turning in a FULL CIRCLE right (2 counts each)
     Arms: Clap once for each Break.

(8 counts)   **Kick "Cool"—4** (2 counts each)
     Arms: Swing arms side to side right, left, right, left, ending each swing with a finger-snap.

Body benefits: neck, shoulders and legs

Practice 2 times

PACING PATTERN

LEARN THESE STEPS:

One-Step "Backstroke"

(directions for one right-and-left set)

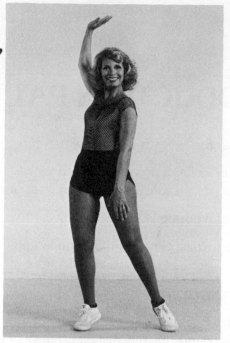

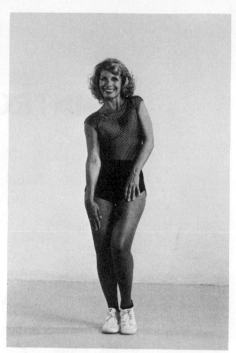

Count: 1   Begin with weight on left foot, hands loosely resting on front of thighs. Step **right** foot to right side as right arm begins circling forward and up to overhead with palm out.

2   Pull **left** foot in to right foot as right arm continues circling back and down with palm out, to end with hand loosely resting on front of thigh.

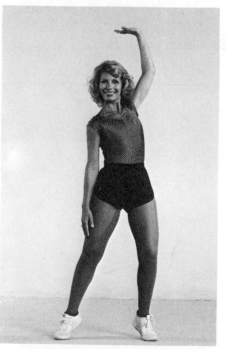

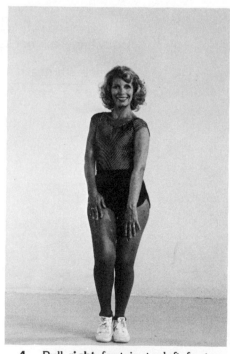

3   Step **left** foot to left side as left arm begins circling forward and up to overhead with palm out.

4   Pull **right** foot in to left foot as left arm continues circling back and down with palm out, to end with hand loosely resting on front of thigh.

146

Break Slow

(directions for one)

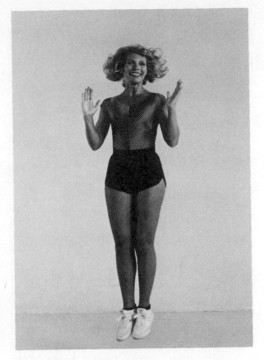

Jump up, keeping feet together.
1. As feet **land,** clap hands close in front of chest, keeping knees re-
2. laxed, then add a small **bounce.**

PACING PATTERN

(8 counts)   **One-Step "Backstroke"—2** right-and-left sets (4 counts each set)
      Arms: Backstroke 4 times, alternating right and left.

(4 counts)   **Break Slow—2** (2 counts each)
      Arms: Clap once for each Break.

Body benefits: arms, waist and legs

Practice 2 times.

RAINBOW PATTERN

LEARN THESE STEPS:

Four-Step "Rainbows"

(directions for right)

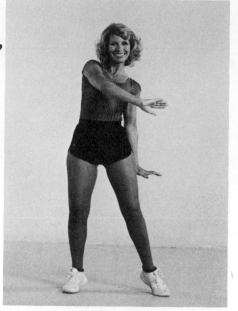

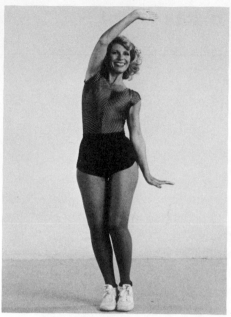

Count: 1   Begin with feet together, weight on left foot, arms down at sides with wrists flexed back. Step **right** foot to right side as right arm begins circling across body and around *clockwise.*

2   Pull **left** foot in to right foot as right arm continues circling across body and up.

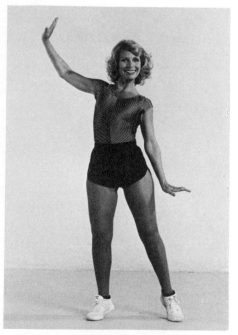

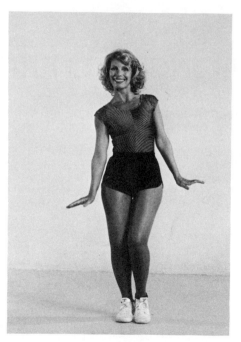

4   Pull **left** foot in to right foot as right arm continues circling to
5,6   end down at side. REPEAT
7,8   THESE 4 STEPS, circling right arm again, and ending with arms down at side, wrists flexed back.

(Reverse to do moving left, circling left arm *counterclockwise.*)

3   Step **right** foot to right side as right arm continues circling out and around.

Break Slow

(directions for one)

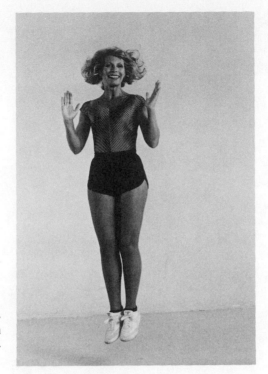

Jump up, keeping feet together.
1   As feet **land,** clap hands close in front of chest, keeping knees re-
2   laxed, then add a small **bounce.**

RAINBOW PATTERN

(16 counts)   **Four-Step "Rainbow"—to the right, to the left** (8 counts each)
Arms: Right arm stretches across, up, and around 2 times when moving right; left arm stretches across, up, and around 2 times when moving left.

(4 counts)   **Break Slow—2** (2 counts each)
Arms: Clap once for each Break.

Body benefits: arms, waist and legs

Practice 2 times.

LONG PACING PATTERN

LEARN THESE STEPS:

One-Step "Backstroke"

(directions for one right and left set)

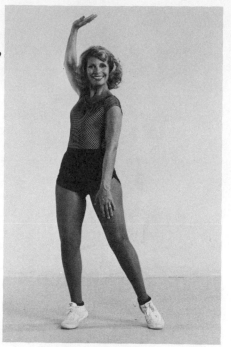

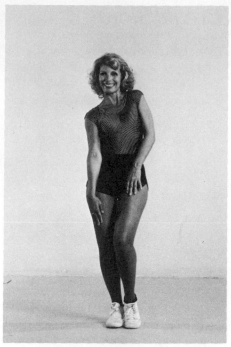

Count: 1   Begin with weight on left foot, hands loosely resting on front of thighs. Step **right** foot to right side as right arm begins circling forward and up to overhead with palm out.

2   Pull **left** foot in to right foot as right arm continues circling back and down with palm out, to end with hand loosely resting on front of thigh.

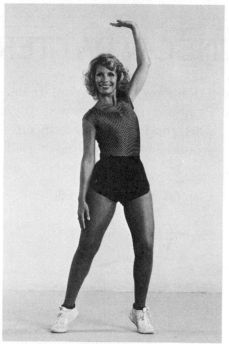

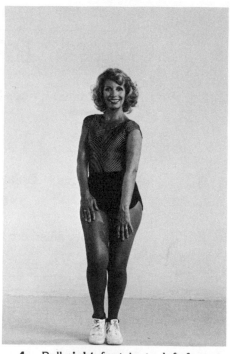

3   Step **left** foot to left side as left arm begins circling forward and up to overhead with palm out.

4   Pull **right** foot in to left foot as left arm continues circling back and down with palm out to end with hand loosely resting on front of thigh.

Break Slow

(directions for one)

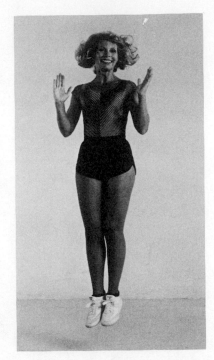

Jump up, keeping feet together.
1 As feet **land,** clap hands close in front of chest, keeping knees re-
2 laxed, then add a small **bounce.**

LONG PACING PATTERN

(8 counts)   **One-Step "Backstroke"—2** right-and-left sets (4 counts each set)
   Arms: Backstroke 4 times, alternating right and left.

(4 counts)   **Break Slow—2** (2 counts each)
   Arms: Clap once for each Break.

(8 counts)   **One-Step "Backstroke"—2** right-and-left sets (4 counts each set)
   Arms: Backstroke 4 times, alternating right and left.

(8 counts)   **Break Slow—4** turning in a FULL CIRCLE right
   Arms: Clap once for each Break.

Body benefits: arms, waist and legs

Practice 2 times.

HI-HO-SILVER PATTERN

LEARN THESE STEPS:

Four-Step "Lasso"

(directions for right)

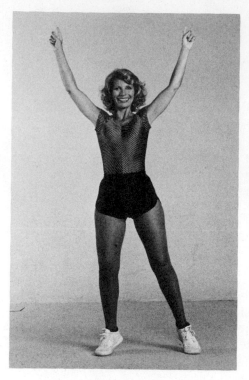

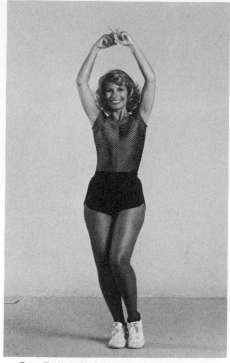

Count:

1 Begin with weight on left foot, arms extended overhead with elbows relaxed, hands in loose fists and index fingers pointing up. Step **right** foot to right side as arms begin twirling inward, making a medium circle overhead.

2 Pull **left** foot in to right foot as arms finish making a medium circle overhead. Repeat THREE MORE TIMES.

3,4
5,6
7,8

(Reverse to do moving left.)

Break Slow

(directions for one)

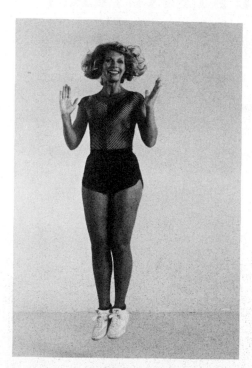

1 Jump up, keeping feet together. As feet **land,** clap hands close in front of chest, keeping knees relaxed, then add a small **bounce.**

2

One-Step "Lasso"

(directions for one right-and-left set)

1 Begin with feet together, weight on left foot, arms extended overhead with elbows relaxed, hands in loose fists and index fingers pointing up. Step **right** foot to right side as arms begin twirling inward, making a medium circle overhead.

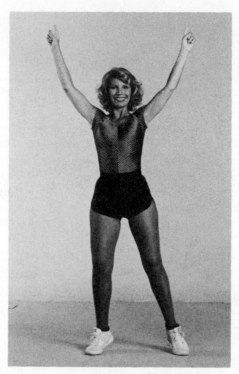

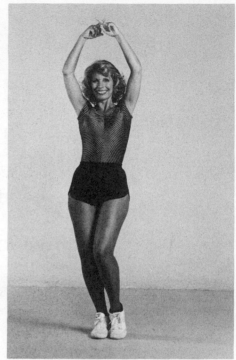

2 Pull **left** foot in to right foot as arms finish making a medium circle overhead.

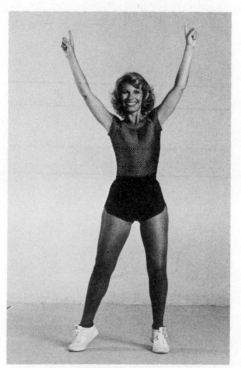

3 Step **left** foot to left side as arms begin twirling inward, making a medium circle overhead.

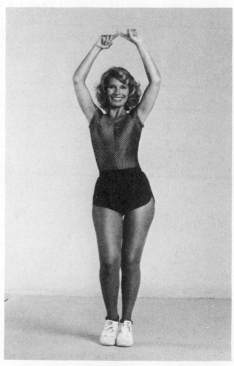

4 Pull **right** foot in to left foot as arms finish making a medium circle overhead.

(continued)

HI-HO-SILVER PATTERN

(16 counts) **Four-Step "Lasso"—to the right, to the left** (8 counts each)
Arms: Overhead, arms twirl inward 4 times for each Four-Step.

(4 counts) **Break Slow—2** (2 counts each)
Arms: Clap once for each Break.

(12 counts) **One-Step "Lasso"—Do 3** right-and-left sets (4 counts each)
Arms: Overhead, arms twirl inward for each One-Step.

(4 counts) **Break Slow—2**
Arms: Clap once for each Break.

Body benefits: arms, waist and legs

Practice 2 times.

HALLELUJAH PATTERN

LEARN THESE STEPS:

Knee-Lifts Hopping "Shoot-Up"

(directions for two)

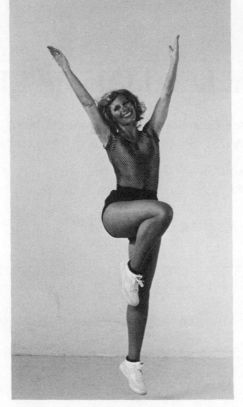

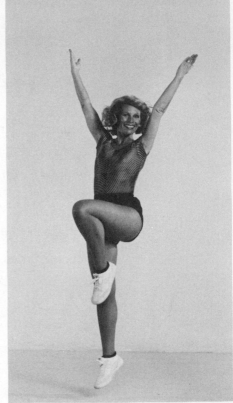

Count:
Begin with feet together, arms close in front of chest. Hop on
1 **left** foot as you lift right knee and arms shoot up overhead.
2 Bounce **both feet** together as arms pull in close in front of chest.

1 Hop on **right** foot as you lift left knee and arms shoot up over
2 head. Then bounce **both feet** together as arms pull in close in front of chest.

Break Slow

(directions for one)

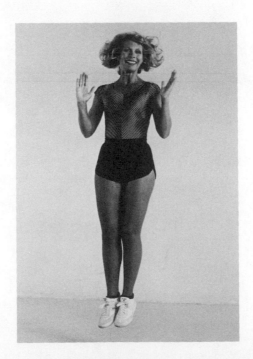

Jump up, keeping feet together.
1 As feet **land,** clap hands close in front of chest, keeping knees re-
2 laxed, then add a small **bounce.**

(continued)

HALLELUJAH PATTERN

(8 counts)   **Knee-Lifts Hopping—4** (2 counts each)
          Arms: Shoot up and pull in for each Knee-Lift Hopping.

(4 counts)   **Break Slow—2** (2 counts each)
          Arms: Clap once for each Break.

Body benefits: arms, waist, hips, seat, legs, front of thighs and back of thighs

Practice 2 times.

FINALE PATTERN

LEARN THESE STEPS:

Break Slow

(directions for one)

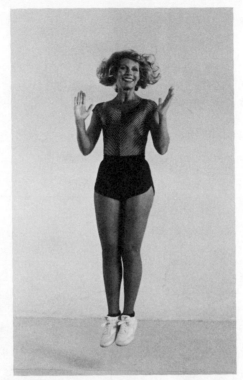

Count: Jump up, keeping feet together.
1   As feet **land,** clap hands close in
     front of chest, keeping knees re-
2   laxed, then add a small **bounce.**

Break "Anchored"

(directions for one)

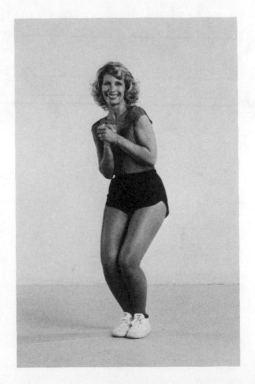

     Jump up, keeping feet together.
1   As feet **land,** clap hands close in
     front of chest, keeping knees re-
     laxed, and hold this position.

(continued)

FINALE PATTERN

(8 counts)   **Break Slow—4** turning in a FULL CIRCLE right (2 counts each)
         Arms: Clap once for each Break.

(1 count)   **Break "Anchored"—1**
         Arms: Clap once and hold

Body benefits: Emotional! This pattern ends the dance and will leave you feeling successful and emotionally high!

Practice 2 to 100 times. (Practice makes perfect!)

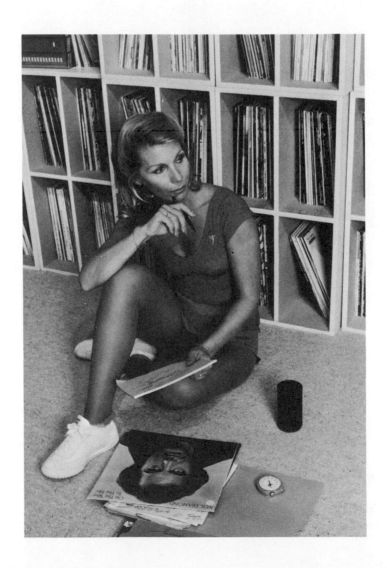

Now that you've learned the new patterns, review the following patterns from Chapter Four:

50s PATTERN

(16 counts) **Two-Step "Stroll-It"—to the right, to the left, to the right, to the left** (4 counts each)
Arms: Close ready-to-jog position; clap on each 4th count.

(8 counts) **Jog "Wild"—8** turning in a FULL CIRCLE right
Arms: Extended overhead, arms sway side to side vigorously.

(8 counts) **Kick "Cool"—4** (2 counts each)
Arms: Swing hands from shoulder to shoulder, right, left, right, left. End each swing with a finger-snap.

Review one time

POLKA PATTERN

(16 counts) **Polka Combo—to the right, to the left** (8 counts each)
Arms: Push-pull arms on each heel-toe, then hold arms in ready-to-jog position.

(2 counts) **Jump/Half-Turn—1** (to end facing the *rear*)
Arms: Ready-to-jog position

(2 counts) **Break Fast—2** (facing the *rear*) (one count each)
Arms: Clap once for each Break.

(2 counts) **Jump/Half-Turn—1** (to end facing the *front*)
Arms: Ready-to-jog position

(2 counts) **Break Fast—2** (facing the *front*)
Arms: Clap once for each Break.

(8 counts) **Knee-Lifts Hopping—4** (2 counts each)
Arms: Hands on hips with alternating shoulder lifts

Review one time

THERE'S NO STOPPING YOU! PATTERN

(6 counts)   **Thigh Rock Double—3** (2 counts each)
    Arms: "Stop Hand"—Single push left forward for 2 counts, right forward for 2 counts, then left forward for 2 counts

(2 counts)   **Break Fast—2** (one count each)
    Arms: Clap hands once for each Break.

(6 counts)   **Thigh Rock Double—3**
    Arms: "Stop Hand"—Single push left forward for 2 counts, then right forward for 2 counts, then left forward for 2 counts

(2 counts)   **Break Fast—2**
    Arms: Clap hands once for each Break.

(4 counts)   **Slides—4** moving to the right
    Arms: Ready-to-jog position

(2 counts)   **Jump Forward, Jump Back—1**
    Arms: Push forward and pull in.

(2 counts)   **Jumping Jack—1**
    Arms: Push out at sides and pull in.

(4 counts)   **Slides—4** moving to the left
    Arms: Ready-to-jog position

(2 counts)   **Jump Forward, Jump Back—1**
    Arms: Push forward and pull in.

(2 counts)   **Jumping Jack—1**
    Arms: Push out at sides and pull in.

Review one time

WORKOUT PATTERN

(32 counts)   **Hustle Jog—4** forward and backward sets (8 counts each) MAKE A SQUARE by turning ¼-turn right each time you hop on left.

       Arms: Ready-to-jog position, clap on each hop.

(16 counts)   **Four-Step "Lift Two Weights"—to right and to left** (8 counts each)

       Arms: Fists shoot up and pull in 4 times each way.

(16 counts)   **Two-Step "Lift One Weight"—to right, to left, to right, to left** (4 counts each)

       Arms: Left arm in close ready-to-jog position; right fist shoots up and pulls in 2 times when moving right. Then right arm in close ready-to-jog position; left fist shoots up and pulls in 2 times when moving left.

Review one time

SWING-OUT PATTERN

(24 counts)   **Cha-Cha "Swing-Out"—3** (8 counts each)

       Arms: Swing arms out at sides to overhead, then swing down to cross in front of chest 2 times for each Cha-Cha.

(4 counts)   **Jump/Half-Turn—2** (to make a complete turn to the left)

       Arms: Ready-to-jog position

(4 counts)   **Break Slow—2** (2 counts each)

       Arms: Clap once for each Break.

(24 counts)   **Slide 'n' Step Back "Swing-Out"—6** (4 counts each) alternating to the right and left

       Arms: Swing arms out at sides to overhead then swing down to cross in front of chest once for each Slide 'n' Step Back.

(4 counts)   **Jump/Half-Turn—2** (to make a complete turn to the left)

       Arms: Ready-to-jog position

(4 counts)   **Break Slow—2**

       Arms: Clap once for each Break.

Review one time

NOW YOU'RE READY TO DANCE!

Aerobic Dance:

"Hooked on Classics"

INTRODUCTION PATTERN—do once
  (Wait 3 counts before starting)
  Shoulder Rolls Single—right and left
  Wait 3 counts
  Shoulder Rolls Single—right and left
  Wait 3 counts
  Shoulder Rolls Single—6, alternating right and left
  Break Slow—4 in a FULL CIRCLE turning right (2 counts each)
  Kick "Cool"—4 (2 counts each)

50s PATTERN—do once
  Two-Step "Stroll-It"—right, left, right, left (4 counts each)
  Jog "Wild"—8 in a FULL CIRCLE turning right
  Kick "Cool"—4 (2 counts each)

PACING PATTERN—do once
  One-Step "Backstroke"—2 right-and-left sets
  Break Slow—2

POLKA PATTERN—do once
  Polka Combo—right and left (8 counts each)
  Jump/Half-Turn—1 to face rear
  Break Fast—2
  Jump/Half-Turn—1 to face front
  Break Fast—2
  Knee-Lifts Hopping—4 (2 counts each)

PACING PATTERN—do once

RAINBOW PATTERN—do two times
  Four-Step "Rainbows"—right and left (8 counts each)
  Break Slow—2 (2 counts each)

PACING PATTERN—do once

THERE'S NO STOPPING YOU! PATTERN—do once
  Thigh Rock Double—3
  Break Fast—2
  Thigh Rock Double—3
  Break Fast—2
  Slides—4 moving to the right

Jump Forward, Jump Back—1
Jumping Jack—1
Slides—4 moving to the left
Jump Forward, Jump Back—1
Jumping Jack—1

PACING PATTERN—do once

WORKOUT PATTERN—do once
Hustle Jog—4 forward and backward sets (8 counts each) TO MAKE A
    SQUARE
Four-Step "Lift Two Weights"—right and left (8 counts each)
Two-Step "Lift One Weight"—right, left, right, left (4 counts each)

LONG PACING PATTERN—do once
One-Step "Backstroke"—2 right-and-left sets
Break Slow—2
One-Step "Backstroke"—2 right-and-left sets
Break Slow—4 in a FULL CIRCLE turning right

POLKA PATTERN—do once

HI-HO-SILVER PATTERN—do once
Four-Step "Lasso"—right and left (8 counts each)
Break Slow—2
One-Step "Lasso"—3 right-and-left sets
Break Slow—2

POLKA PATTERN—do once

SWING-OUT PATTERN—do once
Cha-Cha "Swing-Out"—3 (8 counts each)
Jump/Half-Turn—2
Break Slow—2
Slide 'n' Step Back "Swing-Out"—6 (alternating to right and to left; 4
    counts each)
Jump/Half-Turn—2
Break Slow—2

HALLELUJAH PATTERN—do once
Knee-Lifts Hopping "Shoot-Up"—4 (2 counts each)
Break Slow—2

SWING-OUT PATTERN—do once

THERE'S NO STOPPING YOU! PATTERN—do once

WORKOUT PATTERN—do once

(continued)

FINALE PATTERN—do once
   Break Slow—4 in a FULL CIRCLE turning right
   Break "Anchored"—1

Important: Immediately take your working heart rate as you listen to the
APPLAUSE . . . APPLAUSE . . . APPLAUSE!

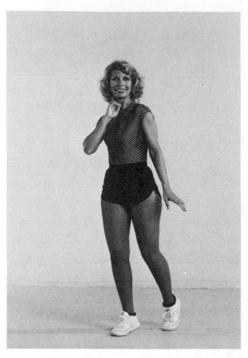 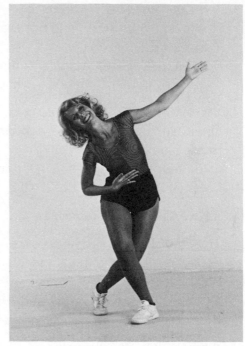

6

Eating for a Trim Life

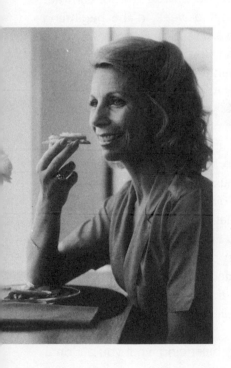

Exercise and eating get equal attention in my aerobic lifestyle because there's a simple, inescapable concept at work: your body is a machine that takes in fuel and if you don't use that fuel, you're going to store it as FAT. Thus, when it comes to losing weight or maintaining a desired weight level, my theme has long been that good eating patterns *and* aerobic exercise are the winning combination.

To me, however, this ongoing motivation so many of us have to get trim and stay trim—in a *healthy* way—certainly doesn't mean "going on a diet." I've never been on a diet (though I was once 20 pounds over my desired weight) because I know I could never live with one. Eating is a pleasurable part of life and I love the tastes and textures of so many different foods that I'm not about to jeopardize that fun by forcing myself to follow a strict diet.

Actually, I did try the Stillman Diet one day back in 1971. Neil wanted to lose weight, as did Mommy and my sister Debra, so we all decided to start together. I remember saying, "You people are crazy," but I wanted to help motivate Neil, who wasn't about to try a diet unless I did it with him. We started the diet and that night, to keep our minds off eating, Neil took us out to a movie. Once we were seated he said he was going to get us some popcorn, but I reminded him we couldn't have anything like *that*. Good ol' Neil then said, "That's ridiculous. Who can watch a movie without eating popcorn?" Thus ended our stab at dieting.

One reason virtually all diets ultimately fail to work for nearly all people is that a strict diet plan makes unreasonable demands. Usually when you're on a diet, all you think about is food, which makes temptation harder and harder to resist with every passing hour . . . or day. I also don't believe that you're going to see any permanent change that will make you feel that losing weight is worth giving things up for.

Instead of giving you a strict diet plan, I'm going to emphasize a positive, realistic approach that can motivate you to give away all the fad diet books you might now own. Basically, I believe in simply eating a little better every week, month by month. By modifying your eating patterns slightly, you can control calories and introduce better nutrition in a gentle way that fits your style FOR THE REST OF YOUR LIFE. Besides, it's much more fun to think about what to eat—moderately and at times sparingly—as opposed to focusing on what *not* to eat. I want to inspire you to devise an eating program that you can *realistically* work into your daily life, not one based on the latest best-selling diet that may not suit your tastes, will prove too restrictive, and could even be dangerous.

You can't expect to change lifelong eating patterns overnight, but you can do it *gradually* by incorporating better habits and nutritional good sense (and, yes, *some* willpower). I take the same approach here that I do with people beginning an aerobic fitness program. We start with a bare-minimum goal and we improve from there in small, one-step-at-a-time changes. So, I want three or four days of improved eating from you as we strive for slimmer eating patterns, but I'll compromise on two days a week in the beginning (and even *one* day if your current eating plan is a disaster). Soon you should find that a third day of semi-sensible eating comes easily, and through continued moderation you can make the gradual changes that don't require a lot of willpower but will result in a happier, healthier lifestyle.

I don't believe in giving things up completely when it comes to eating. Even if some of your favorite foods just drip with calories, that's still too much pleasure to forfeit for the rest of your life. So, if your mouth waters at the thought of hot fudge sundaes, it's unrealistic to say that you're never going to have one again. Instead, decide to treat yourself once every two weeks instead of every week. That's a start in the right direction.

My approach also means that I'm going to let you go to a local fast-food franchise once or twice a week *if* that's what you enjoy doing. Don't feel guilty —just go and enjoy!—but keep those meals in perspective. As I've told my Aerobic Dancing instructors, "My 'recommended nutrition allowance' is to eat super-healthy meals *most of the time,* and then an occasional fast-food taste treat is fun and fine." This is what I believe ... a gentle, we're-only-human approach.

Another of my eating mottos is: *Balance.* By balancing what you eat on a daily or weekly basis, you have the freedom to splurge occasionally as long as you compensate. This approach doesn't mean you have to start eating only "health" foods, or boring foods, or follow a menu you don't like. Nor does it require extra money or creative talent—just some good common sense, and that's free!

On the following pages are dozens of hints about eating, nutrition, and weight control that you can try to work into your daily life in the coming years

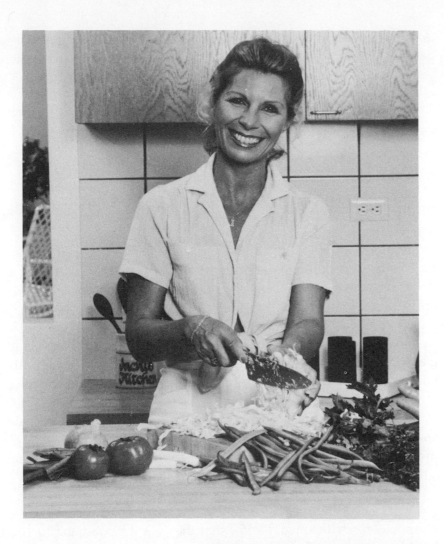

—ideally, without any great deprivation to body or soul. These are hints that have helped me maintain a trim weight in a profession where every calorie saved counts.

I'll talk in this chapter about how I motivate myself to eat semi-sensibly to help achieve my weight goals, but ultimately you must motivate yourself to reach your goal . . . I can't do it for you. So begin now! Scan the healthy hints that follow and choose two as a gift to yourself. Then when you've grown accustomed to these two and they fit into your daily eating patterns without making you feel cheated, why not choose two more? That's how I've adopted healthier eating habits since the early 1970s.

My friend Deborah Szekely, owner of the Golden Door Fitness Spa, reflected my philosophy about eating when she said, "Loving food is part of loving life." I know that I can't think of food just as fuel, or else I'd be looking forward to the year 2000 when all we may need is a handful of pills every day.

Food is like a loving friend, but I also know that it's more interesting to have a variety of friends. So think of your new eating patterns as a chance to acquire interesting new friends who will help you look better and feel better in the years to come. Whether you're fat or thin or just right, view these patterns as a lifetime balancing opportunity. Strive to eat a bit better each year—and don't forget: add more action to every year!

EIGHT TO GET YOU STARTED

1. If you love to eat, your eating opportunities can be more frequent or will last longer if you eat lower-calorie foods.

2. If you can't cut *out* high-calorie foods, cut *down* the amount you eat—and the frequency.

3. Before you start eating, decide upon the *right* amount to eat and then don't eat what's *left.* (Where do you want to store your leftovers: in your refrigerator or on your hips?)

4. One way to help curb your appetite before lunch or dinner is to have a glass of tomato juice—only 25 calories in a half cup. (Since both tomato juice and V-8 are high in sodium, you might want to try low-sodium versions.)

5. When you eat, do it slowly and savor the experience. I was once the fastest eater in my family, but I've gradually slowed down so that I can enjoy my food more, especially since I'm eating less. I cut my food into small pieces and I almost always put my fork down between bites.

6. Avoid using food as a comfort when you're anxious, sad, bored, angry, disappointed, or fatigued. I know that this is a difficult habit to shed, since food is a great pacifier, but now's the time to at least start *thinking* about how you might adjust.

7. By the same token, when you want to celebrate, food shouldn't always be used as THE reward. A joyful part of life is going to a nice restaurant to celebrate a special occasion, or to attend a buffet party, and food is a natural part of the festivities. Just remember *moderation.* Living life in all ways should also be part of your self-reward system, and the rewards can be as simple as a long, peaceful walk or a quiet evening spent reading a romantic novel or the latest non-fiction best seller.

8. Instead of trying various weight-control programs devised by others, use this book to help create your OWN program.

BEST BETS FOR THE 100-CALORIES CLUB

One of the most interesting discoveries I made during a visit to the Golden Door was a table that listed foods in 100-calorie portions. I had no idea there could be such a diversity of options in the servings offered. I've since compiled a list of foods that I commonly enjoy in my diet and the amounts I can eat to spend about 100 calories that I've *earned* through exercise (such as the equivalent of a brisk 15-minute walk).

Apple: 1 medium
Banana: 1 medium
Broccoli (fresh): 2½ cups
Butter: 1 tablespoon
Cantaloupe: 1 small
Celery: 14 large stalks
Cheese (Muenster): 1-ounce slice
Chicken (white meat): ½ cup
Cottage cheese (low-fat): 10
   tablespoons
Egg (large): 1¼
Green beans (fresh): 3 cups
Hot dog (with bun): ⅓
Lettuce (romaine): 20 leaves (8″)
Mayonnaise: 1 tablespoon
Milk (non-fat): 1 cup
Muffin (bran): 1 small
Mushrooms (fresh): 5 cups

Orange: 1 large
Orange juice (fresh): 1 cup
Peanut butter: 1 tablespoon
Pear: 1 medium
Pineapple (raw): 1½ cups
Plums: 4 medium
Popcorn (plain): 2½ cups (or 2
   tablespoons of peanuts!)
Potato (baked): 1 small
Raisins: ¼ cup
Rice (natural brown, cooked): ½ cup
RyKrisp: 4
Spinach (fresh, trimmed): 4 cups
Strawberries (fresh): 2 cups
Tomatoes: 3 medium
Tuna (packed in water): 3 ounces
Watermelon: 2 cups
Zucchini (fresh): 5 cups!

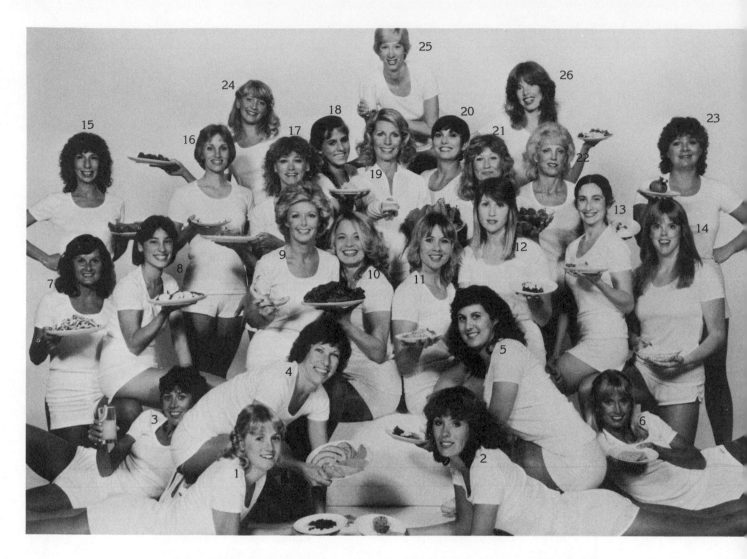

Holding 100-calorie portions of some of my favorite foods are the following friends and colleagues:

1. Raisins: Cecelia Maron-Puntarelli
2. Muffin: April Schauer
3. Orange juice: Janci Farwell
4. Cantaloupe: Teckla Armantrout
5. Mayonnaise: Sue Satuloff
6. RyKrisp: Rochelle Munson
7. Mushrooms: Pat Herold
8. Zucchini: Karen House
9. Banana: Sally Levy
10. Spinach: Pat Sramek
11. Tuna: Rita Teel
12. Butter: Nancy Gitto
13. Cheese: Shelly Deutsch
14. Popcorn: Sherri Parrish
15. Tomatoes: Phyllis Stein
16. Cottage Cheese: Adelle Masto
17. Green beans: Anita Goldman
18. Rice: Stacey Clinesmith
19. Hot dog: Guess Who?
20. Lettuce: Janis "JJ" Johnson
21. Strawberries: Deborah Maron
22. Egg: Marilyn Darnell
23. Potato: Nancy Roth
24. Broccoli: Beverly Pearson
25. Milk: Vicki Neschke
26. Chicken: Angela Gomes

NUTRITION NOTES

While the focus in this chapter is on calorie-saving hints and how to incorporate them into a realistic eating plan, we certainly can't overlook the importance of nutrition in a healthy aerobic lifestyle. I'm not going to give you a course in nutrition here, but I do want to point out some guidelines that have helped me adopt better eating habits over the years.

1. If you're aerobically active and follow a well-balanced eating plan, you should get ample vitamins and minerals in your food without having to take supplements. The key is to exercise enough every week so you can consume a sufficient amount of food to meet your vitamin and mineral needs while still maintaining a desired weight.

2. By a "balanced" diet, I mean eating adequate servings from the four basic food groups:
   - Breads and cereals (with an emphasis on whole grains).
   - Fruits and vegetables (especially eaten fresh, either raw or steamed).
   - Fish, poultry, and meats (minimizing red meat consumption and substituting other protein sources such as beans, seeds, nuts, and tofu).
   - Dairy products (stressing non-fat or low-fat varieties).

3. Since I want to keep my iron reserves high to ensure a high physical work capacity, I make sure I eat iron-rich foods, particularly eggs, whole-grain bread, lean meats, raisins and dark leafy vegetables such as spinach.

4. Potassium is particularly important for active people, so I don't forget my daily orange juice. Other good potassium sources are potatoes, grapefruit, bananas, raisins, and milk.

5. Our body's need for calcium doesn't end when we stop growing, as evidenced by the calcium deficiencies which can show up when we're older, either in the form of osteoporosis (pitted and brittle bones) or osteomalacia (soft bones). Our bones remain biologically active throughout our lives, so our total daily intake of calcium should be at least 800–1000 mg a day (and higher for teenagers and pregnant or breastfeeding women). Low-fat milk and yogurt are healthy sources of calcium (supplying from 298 to 345 mg a cup) along with those trusty standbys, spinach and broccoli. Cheese is also high in calcium, and if you should happen to consume an entire 14-inch pizza, it might ease your guilt to know that you've at least satisfied your daily requirement of calcium.

6. Fiber, of course, is crucial to a well-functioning body and is an important element in helping the body absorb other foods. I choose from fresh fruits, fresh vegetables, bran discs, bran muffins, and bran cereal to meet my fiber needs.

7. If you're active, your eating plan should also include sufficient complex carbohydrates such as pastas, whole-grain breads, potatoes and brown rice. This will maintain the glycogen stored in your muscles and will help prevent early fatigue or cramps as you participate in your favorite sport.

8. One of the best changes I've made in my eating habits in recent years—in terms of better nutrition—has been a simple one: switching from instant white rice to brown rice. I have to cook it 30 minutes, but it's a more natural food, it's higher in fiber, and it tastes terrific. So why waste your precious calories on white rice?

9. Needless to say, any nutritious eating plan includes cutting down on fatty foods and reducing your overall intake of saturated fats.

SALT-PINCHING SUGGESTIONS

There's an important controversy going on these days between nutritionists who advise us to cut down on salt to help prevent high blood pressure and experts in hypertension who seriously doubt that reducing salt intake is necessary for most people. Yet, even if salt is given a reprieve, I'm heeding the advice of my medical consultant, Dr. John Boyer, who said, "The American diet is outrageously high in salt and almost all of us would benefit by decreasing our sodium intake. We do not have to be on a salt-free diet, but we certainly should follow a sodium-restricted diet." Here are some ways I'm working to lower my salt and sodium intake—gradually and gently—to keep it closer to the recommended levels.

—I always taste first, then salt if needed. (At least that's *one* bite without extra salt.)

—I'm *trying* to leave the salt shaker off the table at dinner.

—Neil and I have eliminated many once-favored salty foods from our regular diet, such as chips, sausages, snack crackers, sardines, and pork chops.

—Fool your tongue's "need" for salt by substituting herbs and spices when cooking. Some of the tastier ones are tarragon, dill, oregano, paprika, and ginger. Other allies are curry powder, garlic powder, and pepper.

—Read food labels and become more aware of hidden salt and sodium traps. Here are four "salt heavies" to memorize and avoid: onion and garlic salts, steak sauce, soy sauce, and bouillon cubes.

—High-sodium–containing ingredients in recipes include monosodium glutamate, seasoning salt, baking powder, and baking soda.

—Look for common food products that are now highlighting less salt and fewer sodium-containing ingredients. We will all benefit here in the coming years as the major food companies actively reduce the level of salt in their products and offer a greater variety of salt-free products.

These salt tips may not necessarily apply to you, but lower salt/sodium intake could be important to your spouse or other family members.

SHOPPING STRATEGIES

• I eat *before* I go grocery shopping. Otherwise I'm really tempted to buy something I can eat *while* I'm shopping (like a calorie-filled bag of chips).

• Stick to your grocery list, except when you reach the produce department. Do all your other shopping quickly (aerobic basket-pushing can help burn fat) and finish up in produce. Take time to see what's in season, what looks great, and what appeals to your taste. If you're shopping with children, you may want to start in the fruit and vegetable section, when you're all fresh and eager for the hunt.

• Try to shop from a weekly menu to ensure balanced meals and to keep from running out of basic meal preparations on Wednesday or Thursday night and then opting for a fast-food meal. (It's best to shop at least twice a week to be assured of the freshest foods.)

• Learn to understand food labels so that you're better aware of the calories and relative content of sodium, sugar, and non-nutritive additives in the foods you buy. Also:

—Just because a packaged food is labeled "low-fat" or "fat-free" or "non-fat" doesn't necessarily mean it's low in calories, and
—Just because a food is labeled "natural" doesn't mean it's low in calories. It means it's low in preservatives.

• I get bored waiting in line at the checkout, so to keep my eyes off the candy displays, I pick up a magazine I want to buy and begin reading it immediately.

COOKING CUES

• We all *collect* recipes, but you should read the ingredients first and keep only the ones that are low in calories, healthy, and easy to make. Why torture yourself by collecting recipes that feature your high-calorie hang-ups? Also, once you've collected these great new menu ideas, *use* them!

• Trim all visible fat from meats *before* cooking. This is better for you than trimming after cooking.

• Always remove the skin from chicken. Even when you barbecue it, you can keep the meat moist by marinating it in low-calorie Italian dressing for 30 to 60 minutes before cooking. You'll love the taste!

- With recipes where fat becomes a part of the liquid (and cooks into the liquid), cook the required ingredients a day ahead of time and put them into the refrigerator. Then you can remove the hardened fat that surfaces on the food before it surfaces on your body. This is also a great visual reminder that some recipes shouldn't be consumed too frequently. (A tablespoon of congealed fat, removed from the top of cooked stews or meaty soups, represents 125 calories conquered.)

- When recipes call for certain ingredients, I'm learning I can use low-calorie substitutes without affecting the appeal of the final product. For instance, I use low-fat yogurt instead of sour cream in one of my favorite dishes, a crustless broccoli quiche, and I use low-calorie mozzarella cheese instead of higher-calorie cheddar.

- Nearly all of us need to eat more fresh vegetables—raw or cooked. Be careful not to overcook, since this lowers the nutrient content.

- Here's one way that I encourage healthier eating around my house. Every now and then I put a whole chicken in a pot of water, then let it boil as I go about my other work. After it's done and cools, I remove the skin and throw away the fat that has congealed on the broth. (I later make a homemade soup using the broth.) Next I put the whole chicken in a casserole dish and store it in the refrigerator where it's ready for lunch, and for those recipes that call for "one cup of cooked chicken."

- I try to plan ahead in my shopping in order to avoid leftovers, but it's not always easy to buy the right amount for a single meal. So what I do is freeze our leftovers as soon as I serve our portions at dinner. This keeps us from having unnecessary seconds and saves me from being tempted by easily accessible leftovers the next day.

- No need to give up cooking with butter and cream; just use *less* butter and cream and make lighter sauces.

BREAKFAST IDEAS

Your body has been resting all night and you want to begin your day "feelin' good," right? An exercise routine (my Everyday Eights!) will give you a terrific start, but don't overlook the importance of a nutritious breakfast to provide the right kind of energy all morning. Try to include fruit, protein, and something from the grain group.

I have half a container of fruit yogurt for breakfast and I've trained myself to believe that this is a treat because I sample all flavors and I change from day to day. Also, I have a small glass of orange juice and I enjoy a cup of coffee, usually my only caffeine of the day, diluted with one-quarter cup of non-fat milk.

Here are other thoughts I have about breakfast:

• Personally, I don't enjoy special breakfast drinks, even if they are terrific for protein. It seems as though I'm eating more if I eat the ingredients separately. And, when they are liquefied in one tall glass, the eating experience is over too quickly.

• When I travel, I sometimes treat myself to dry cereal, but always a high-fibered brand. I add fruit instead of sugar to make it taste sweeter.

• I'm not endorsing no-breakfast mornings, but I feel it's better to skip breakfast if it's going to be a "bad" breakfast, such as a doughnut and coffee. Eating a breakfast like this will give you a low, depressed feeling later in the morning—just when you ought to be feeling bright and energetic.

• If you're a working person and you can't manage to eat breakfast before you leave home, then establish the "take-out pattern." Take yogurt, cottage cheese, or a hard-boiled egg *out* to work and eat when you have a few minutes to really enjoy it. This will also help you avoid the doughnut-for-breakfast trap at work.

LUNGING THROUGH LUNCH

When I'm working at home, I rarely sit down and have a typical lunch; I'm more of a snacker, at around 11 A.M. and around 3 P.M. (I don't fight it . . . that's just the way I am!)

Since I normally have my breakfast around 6 A.M., I'm ready for a quick but nutritious snack by late morning—perhaps a granola bran cereal that I eat dry, or a bran muffin. My midafternoon snack will include either some fresh fruit or a small amount of low-fat cottage cheese. Sometimes I pull out a bran disc and top it with a little mayonnaise and a tomato slice.

If I go out for lunch, I almost always order a salad. Tossed salad and spinach salad are my favorites, with vinegar and oil or the house dressing if it's light. Tuna or chicken salads taste great but are too heavy on the mayonnaise for my eating plan. I also never order a chef's salad because it contains too much processed meat for healthy eating.

Here are some other lunch tips to keep in mind:

• Learn to appreciate the many virtues of low-fat cottage cheese. Here's a food that is (1) low in calories, (2) a source of needed protein and calcium, (3) a good substitute for mayonnaise and sour cream, and (4) a different taste sensation when you whip it in a blender with a little lemon juice. (Since cottage cheese does have a high sodium content, you might want to shop for the unsalted product.)

• I could eat tuna sandwiches every day forever—with extra mayonnaise on the bread—but fortunately I've found I can satisfy my craving by simply adding water-packed, low-salt tuna to my salad. This gives me the great taste of tuna without all those extra calories. (You'll save 250 calories in a seven-ounce can by using water-packed instead of oil-packed tuna.)

• A good way to control portion size is to buy the tiny 3¼ ounce can of tuna. Opening the large can may tempt you to eat more than you need.

• Eating a sandwich open-faced will cut calories, but you can save even more by simply eating half a sandwich. Not only do you eliminate one slice of bread, you avoid eating half the makings.

DELIVER ME TO DINNER

Since many nutritional experts recommend making dinner the *lightest* meal of the day, I'm trying to improve my eating patterns by having salad-only dinners two or three days a week. This doesn't mean, however, that I have a bigger breakfast or a bigger lunch on these days. I simply have an overall light eating day.

Neil and I have gradually changed our tastes over the years to where we can now deemphasize red meat in our diets and not feel deprived. Neil grew up in a meat-and-potatoes family, but he'll now get semi-excited about ordering fish in a restaurant, which is something he never would do when we were first married. This shows again how we can reverse our habits, if only slightly in the beginning.

Basically, this is the order of *healthy* preference in which we have meat:

First, and most frequently, *fish* or *fowl* (chicken and game hens)—never fried, and always without skin or creamy sauces.

Second, *hamburger* (leanest and grilled). Hamburger meat is still my favorite, fixed any way, but especially as a main course hamburger steak. I think this love affair stems from our Air Force days, when we didn't have much money and I was just learning how to cook, so I'd often whip out my trusty copy of *101 Ways to Fix Hamburger.*

Third is *prime ribs* or *steak.* I can save lamb and pork for special occasions, and I've never acquired a taste for veal. We used to have pork chops once a week, but now I fix them only about twice a year as a treat for Neil. He's even half-forgotten how I used to smother them with two cups of croutons mixed with one stick of melted butter, one can of cream of mushroom soup, and chopped onions. Can you imagine!

SENSIBLE SALADS

Since salads are an important part of my daily menu, I'm constantly searching for ways to make them as nutritious and inviting as possible.

• I've found that I can make a hearty salad serve as the main course for dinner by adding such ingredients as:

    —One or two chopped eggs
    —Tuna (water packed)
    —Chicken chunks (without the skin)
    —Grated mozzarella cheese

• When salad is going to be my dinner, my favorite is a Caesar salad. I also have a spinach salad at least once a week, bolstered with fresh zucchini and fresh mushrooms. (Spinach is rich in iron and vitamins A and C, and is *most* nutritious when eaten raw.)

• Add croutons to a salad only when the dinner is light or low in starches or carbohydrates. Otherwise, why add unnecessary calories?

• Most regular bottled dressings contain at least 65 to 70 calories per tablespoon, so go lightly—or switch to tasty reduced-calorie dressings that you like.

• You'll tend to use less dressing if you toss the salad with the dressing. When I first started doing this I'd ask Neil to taste the salad first and if it didn't have enough dressing for him, he could add more. Now he doesn't "need" this extra dressing because he has learned to like a lighter taste.

• If you prefer to make your own salad dressing, find the recipes that require the smallest amount of oil.

• Plan ahead in your shopping so there are always plenty of fresh fixings in your refrigerator to prepare an interesting, tempting salad. When I come back from shopping, I set aside time to wash all the lettuce and vegetables before storing them in the refrigerator. Then, for two or three days, I can quickly prepare a salad without having to go through the usual cleaning and preparation stage.

SLURPY SOUPS

• Making your own soup from fresh ingredients takes time and planning ahead, but it's worth it to fight off that temptation simply to rely on canned soups, which can be high in sodium.

• When I was growing up I always preferred bean with bacon and cream of mushroom. Now I make (and prefer) chock-full-of-vegetable soups. Or, if there's no time to cook, I'll heat up a light-calorie soup like turkey noodle.

• As much as I *love* soup, the only heavy soups I've eaten in recent years have been eaten out or for a special occasion—and I only have a *cup.* But oh, do I enjoy those creamy soups when I *do* decide to splurge! (Thank goodness I no longer need crumbled crackers on top.)

• On those rare occasions when I have a creamy canned soup at home, I always add non-fat milk for a lighter load of calories. (One cup of skim milk has 85 calories and one cup of whole milk has 150.)

• A cup of light soup before dinner can help curb your appetite in a calming way. Start collecting some tasty water-based recipes and then try having a *cup* as your first course. You'll feel as though you've been eating a lot because your hand is busy making trips to your mouth. And, since hot soup can't be wolfed down, you'll spend more time eating.

RED MEAT RULES

I know you've read about the "dangers" of including too much red meat in your eating plan. Some of you have become vegetarians to avoid the problem, and many of you have cut down your overall consumption of red meat. However, if vegetarianism is not compatible with your taste buds or lifestyle (and it isn't with mine, either), then here are some recommendations:

• Try eating red meat one day less a week each month until you cut down to two or three (or even fewer) red-meat meals per week.

• Try to make better everyday choices. For example, four ounces (a quarter pound) of greasy hamburger has approximately 300 calories, compared to about 90 calories for four ounces of tasty sole.

• Not only are poultry and fish lower in calories than red meat, they have less saturated fat.

- Be aware that you can choose to buy meat lean or fat. So know your grades:

    —*Prime Grade* contains the most fat.

    —*Choice Grade* contains less fat.

    —*Good Grade* contains still less fat.

    (Some markets label hamburger "leanest," or indicate the percentage of fat, so lean toward the leanest!)

DEVILISH DESSERTS

You'll find that I actually don't talk much in this chapter about the evils of excess sugar intake. This reflects the fact that I no longer think much about sugar because I've managed to cut refined sugar almost completely out of my diet. When I'm tempted by something sweet, I mentally think of what it represents in unnecessary and nutritionally-empty calories. This usually makes it easy to tempt my taste buds with something else. I've also found (to my surprise) that if I don't think about desserts every day, I just don't have them. So perhaps the less I say to you about them, the better off we all are? *However,* I do have these thoughts:

- At home, Neil and I rarely have dessert, unless i'ts a really special occasion . . . two or three times a year. We don't even give in to fresh fruit, since dinner is enough for us.

- If a nightly dessert is your custom, save it for later in the evening to spread out your eating enjoyment (and thereby avoid that late-evening snack which would otherwise come in addition to dessert).

- If you like to eat pies, at least cut portions in eighths instead of quarters or sixths.

- When Neil and I go out, we hardly ever order dessert. If we're in the mood, we share one (like the piece of chocolate chip cheesecake we came across recently). If we're with friends who want to indulge, we share two or three different desserts. Having a bite or two of each is better than ordering one whole dessert apiece.

- When celebrating on spontaneous occasions, I want my own dessert and I *won't* share, so there! My three favorites are a chocolate-chip ice cream cone, a hot fudge sundae, and *Bananas Foster*. (If you don't know what this is you are *so* lucky and I'm not giving you the recipe!)

- Seasonal Ideas:

    Winter: Try fresh apple slices sprinkled with cinnamon, nutmeg, and cloves. (If you love a nightly cup of something hot during these cold months, try herb teas.)

    Spring: Fresh berries with cantaloupe, or orange slices with coconut sprinkled on top.

    Summer: Melon balls and grapes mixed together.

    Fall: CHOCOLATE! (Just kidding.) Actually, try cutting out all desserts from Halloween to Thanksgiving and save yourself for the holidays.

- Never eat a dessert you can refuse.

LIQUID LOWDOWNS

- In this day and age, it's easy to overlook the virtues of good old plain water. I'm reminding myself to drink more water throughout the day and I'm feeling better for it, especially when I travel.

- I used to drink up to four diet sodas a day, until I discovered how high they are in sodium and chemicals. I've since cut back and I now remind myself: "Think water instead of soda."

- If you realize that you consume a lot of sodas just because it has become a pattern always to have a can of liquid on standby, better to have a glass of water to gulp.

- Remember that alcohol adds about 200 calories a day to the intake of the average American who drinks.

- Here are some ways to minimize the caloric effects of alcohol:

    —Before your first drink, drink a glass of water with fresh lime or lemon. This makes it easier to *sip* your drink slowly.

    —Avoid sweet alcoholic drinks: they're higher in calories and they taste so good you'll want to drink them faster.

    —Check beer labels and learn to enjoy the taste of the *lightest* ones. (A 12-ounce can of regular beer contains approximately 150 calories, while those in light beer can vary from 70 to 135.)

    —Try to acquire a taste for the light, low-calorie wines which are increasingly available in stores, and which save you about 30 calories per six-ounce glass.

    —Order wine "on the rocks" or spritzed with water, anywhere from a dash to half and half. Connoisseurs may raise their eyebrows, but I enjoy wine this way.

EATING OUT

• When you're going out, one subtle way to curb a tendency to overeat or overindulge is to wear a tight-fitting dress or snug pants. (Wearing a muumuu is to invite dietary disaster!)

• On our way to a restaurant, I'll say to Neil, "I feel like fettuccine and a small salad," or "sole and vegetables," or "two chicken tacos à la carte." By deciding ahead of time, I'm not tempted by the menu and I'm looking forward to what I've decided to have for dinner.

• When you're going to a restaurant that tends to serve large portions, consider sharing a meal.

• Neil and I are trying to eat more sensibly all the time, so very often I will order only a salad, knowing I can have some of his food. Since he's wonderful about sharing, this helps in two ways: when he orders something that I love, I can at least have a bite or two or three (which is enough to satisfy me) and it cuts down what he's eating. It's also romantic and loving to share.

• As soon as we are seated, I ask that the bread and butter be taken off the table (or not brought to the table), because I know I will just eat it. At a Mexican restaurant, I'm *thinking about* banning tortilla chips and salsa from our table.

• Try eating an appetizer as your *main* course, but then don't fill up by eating all the bread on the table!

• Artichokes are delicious and take a long time to eat, so why not order them as an appetizer that continues into being part of your main course? Just go light on the dip.

• When I order a salad, I ask for dressing on the side so I can control my destiny. I keep in mind that one tablespoon of regular French dressing contains 100 calories as compared to 41 calories when I mix one teaspoon of oil with one teaspoon of vinegar.

• One of my newer taste treats is pasta, which is *not* that fattening as long as you don't layer it with heavy meat sauces. Pasta is delicious plain, but you also ought to try it primavera style. When you're having any kind of pasta, you don't need croutons on your salad and you don't need garlic bread. My friends say, "You can't eat pasta without garlic bread," but I ask them, "Where's your willpower?"

• Restaurants are beginning to offer a variety of entrees with lighter sauces (using less butter and cream), so ask your waiter for more "saucy" information.

• When ordering a steak, ask for the smallest cut offered. Eat half and either share the other half with your partner or take it home and freeze it.

• The next time you order a baked potato, try my tactic: ask the waiter to scoop out the inside of the potato ("out of sight, out of your stomach") and just bring you the baked skin. Then you're free to add a bit of sour cream or butter and chives so that you get that same wonderful taste but with fewer overall calories. Potato skins are available in many restaurants today, especially in California, but they come stuffed with crab, creamed tuna, or cheddar cheese with bacon broiled on top. These concoctions taste wonderful, but should obviously be eaten *sparingly,* as a very special treat.

• When I eat Chinese food, I always use chopsticks—because that's another way to enjoy eating while taking a long time to finish.

• When you're really in need of a fast-food fix at the end of a frazzled day, go and enjoy yourself—but cut down on the size of what you order and keep it simple, so you really enjoy one taste at a time. Instead of ordering a bacon cheeseburger, isn't the taste of hamburger itself enough for your senses? How about saving that bacon or cheese for a treat at another time?

TRAVELING TIPS

• On flights, I order a vegetarian meal in advance so I'm not tempted to eat higher-calorie, tired-tasting airline meals.

• I travel with small packages of raisins for a healthy, high-energy snack.

• I also bring along my trusty bran discs (19 calories each) to make sure I get enough fiber every day and because it's a *good* eating habit I can pack in my suitcase to help avoid tasty travel temptations.

• Several hotel chains are making it easier for fitness-conscious travelers to eat right. For example, Hilton coffee shops now offer a "Fitness First" menu which includes calorie counts, and Marriott restaurants have a "Good For You" menu that features low-calorie, low-sodium, and low-cholesterol dishes.

• Many hotels also have built-in fitness opportunities that make it easy for you to balance your *eating* opportunities. Inquire ahead of time, then bring along your workout clothes and bathing suit.

• Just as when I'm home, I keep breakfast simple but nutritious. I order either a Continental breakfast plus skim milk (skipping the rolls and using the butter and jam on my bran discs) or a high-fiber dry cereal with fruit on top. If I feel

I need extra protein, I'll have a soft-boiled egg or scrambled egg, which I put on my bran disc instead of the butter and jam. Balance . . . balance . . . balance!

• I also keep lunch light, and I avoid anything alcoholic. Aside from calorie-control, I want to make sure my body can enjoy an exercise opportunity in the afternoon.

• When I'm ordering from Room Service, I hardly ever look at the menu. I've found that if I ask for what I want, most hotel staffs can usually put it together, even though it's not on the menu.

• On vacation trips, I treat myself to a variety of favorite foods I never have at home, but which I want to taste again. Knowing that I'm going to do this helps me keep the rest of the year in balance.

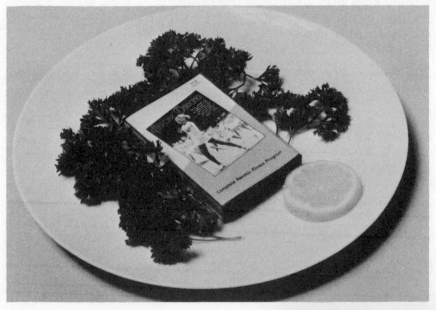

To help you judge the size of a 4-ounce portion, just think of a cassette tape.

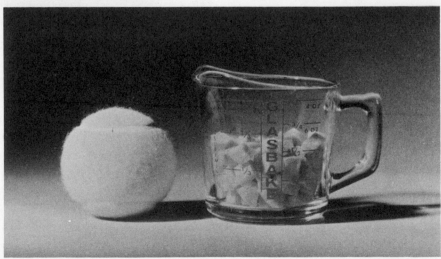

To gauge how much food equals one-half cup, think of a tennis ball.

COPING FROM THANKSGIVING TO NEW YEAR'S

Most all of us must adjust our eating plans around the Holidays, but be kind to yourself: in the spirit of trying to maintain a trim appearance, don't take such a no-to-everything approach that you feel depressed and deprived. Here are some ways I've learned to keep my weight under control in that high-calorie stretch from Thanksgiving through New Year's (which includes my birthday).

• I make sure I'm extra active during the early weeks of December by choreographing a new session of Aerobic Dancing (instead of doing it in November, as I once did).

• Neil and I attend a lot of special luncheons and parties during this time and it's fun to visit because I don't have much time for socializing during the year. So I focus on being with my friends, *not* on the food. I eat lightly (usually salads) but I do join in on desserts (from a bite to half a portion) because that's part of the holiday fun!

• At parties, I never sit or stand next to the food. I also drink at least two glasses of mineral water with lime before I order a white wine spritzer. This helps cut calories.

• I look forward to the special eating days and think about the special foods I'm going to eat on *those* days—like a separate plate of mashed ptoatoes on Thanksgiving, smothered with cream gravy and butter! This makes it easier to be even better on the in-between days.

HOW I DEAL WITH TEMPTATION (FOODS)

I know myself well enough to realize there are certain high-calorie foods that I simply can't resist when they're around. So I ban these foods from my house on the theory, Out of sight, out of my mouth. People who come to visit say, "Good grief, Jacki, you have no food around anywhere." I tell them, "That's right! My plan is to make it inconvenient to overeat. Why should I have something like corn chips around? I would only be tempted to open them and eat them. Then I'd want to fix a dip."

Stripping the house of my temptation foods—things like cheese crackers, peanut butter, corn chips, cookies, M & M's, and yogurt-covered raisins—is essential to my physical well-being, since I work at home most days and I have little willpower when it comes to these foods. I admit that freely! However, I've learned that I simply don't need this stuff to make my day happy.

Here's how I deal with other enticements:

—I *love* hot dogs, so I can never have them in the house or they'd be eaten in short order. When I have one it's a real treat and a meal in itself, not a snack. (My favorite hot dog is Caspers' in California: foot-long, skinny and served on a steamed bun with mustard, relish and wedges of onion and tomato. My second favorite is usually served without a smile on a street corner in New York City.)

—Grease is the word, when it comes to bacon. I love bacon's great taste, but now I use it mainly as a seasoning. I fry a few slices until crispy, drain off the excess grease, then crumble it and bag it to use in salads and in scrambled eggs. This way I'm cutting calories (one slice of bacon represents 80 calories plus fat and salt) and I don't feel cheated!

—Lunch meats are out of my eating plan except for a few slices of salami on pizza about twice a month. This stuff is so easy to eat and not very good for you, so *limit* it!

—Neil and I used to have sausage once a week, but we've cut back to maybe four times a year, when we spontaneously indulge ourselves with a "big" breakfast.

—Duck is fatty, so as much as I enjoy it, we never have it at home and I only order it at a restaurant once or twice a year as a treat.

—Desserts are not allowed in our freezer, but every now and then I find a small container of lemon custard ice cream tucked away in the back. (I love you Neil, but I'd kill you if it were chocolate chip!)

SAYING "NO" DOESN'T HAVE TO MEAN FOREVER

In modifying my own eating habits over the years, I've learned an interesting thing: you don't have to ban certain temptation foods from your house forever. I'll agree, if you can't stop at two or three bites, then you may have to permanently exile things like potato chips, peanuts, crackers, almonds and perhaps pies and cakes (except on special occasions). But as you develop new and healthier eating habits, old patterns are replaced and you'll find that you can eventually bring back certain foods and live with them.

At one point, for example, I couldn't have mayonnaise in the house because it was a high-calorie hang-up at 100 calories—per *tablespoon*! I also had to eliminate bread, since I worked at home most of the time and when I was hungry I always wanted to put something on the bread, like peanut butter and jelly, or tuna and mayonnaise.

Well, I found that without the bread and the mayonnaise around to tempt me, I eventually learned to enjoy my bran muffins and bran discs. Hunger is a great motivator when the taste buds are involved! I followed that pattern for a year or so until I discovered that I could start keeping sourdough English muffins and mayonnaise in the refrigerator without fear. I had acquired a taste for the lower-calorie foods and I could trust myself to eat them as a normal part of my day. It was like winning a battle!

In fact, I can actually look at certain foods I used to eat and wonder *how* I could have loved them so much—things like roasted turkey skin and fried chicken with that yukky skin. Recently, Neil and I both ordered red snapper at a favorite restaurant, except I ordered it broiled and he ordered it fried. When the fish arrived, I wanted a little taste treat (I'm *trying* to avoid all fried foods), so I had a bite of Neil's fried snapper.

"Do you like this, Neil?" I said. "I don't even enjoy that taste anymore."

He tried a bite of my broiled snapper and said, "Yours tastes better to me, too." So you CAN change your tastes!

COPING WITH THE SNACKING URGE

Since indiscriminate snacking—mid-morning, mid-afternoon, and late at night—can undermine the best-intentioned weight-control plan, here are ways I've dealt with this challenge.

• Make sure you're getting enough sleep. When I feel tired I tend to eat more, thinking it will give me more energy. What I need is sleep, not more calories.

• Boredom can lead to constant snacking, so get out of that rut (which doesn't necessarily mean getting out of the house) and entertain yourself with some new project. You might:

      —Start a journal
      —Do needlework
      —Draw, paint, color
      —Play with your pet
      —Write a book
      —Go back to school
      —Try to become more of an expert on something you're interested in
      —Get outside more often for fresh air and exercise.

• Only keep in the house what you have the willpower to resist. Everything else—OUT! Then learn to appreciate the taste and texture of low-calorie foods that can satisfy your snacking urge.

• Enlist your family's support when it comes to eliminating temptation foods from the house. You might tell them: "I'm watching my weight and that means I just can't have any junk food in the house because I'm always the first one to eat it. So here's the plan we have to follow, for my sake at least.

". . . Allison, you're a swimmer and I know you need your nutritious health bars, but they have 400 calories each and I love them as much as you do, so we can't keep them in the pantry anymore. You're going to have to hide them in your room. . . ."

I don't have any children, but when my parents come to visit during the year I have to cope with their habits. For instance, I make Daddy keep his chocolate chip cookies in his bedroom. And when Mommy wants to store any leftovers from our meals in the refrigerator, she has to hide them way in the back.

• If you prefer to save all your leftovers in the refrigerator, then good cooking habits at night (e.g., lower-calorie-type dishes) will help ensure "safer" snacks.

• Junk food is so conveniently tempting that you must compete with that convenience by having healthy snacks already prepared for your raids on the refrigerator—things like celery sticks, fresh mushrooms, cut-up zucchini, and fresh fruit. I also like to keep carrot sticks marinating in reduced-calorie dressing because this gives them a bit more zing.

• Sometimes I just want to *munch,* don't you? If the only thing in the refrigerator or pantry is something "good" for me to eat, then I'll eat it—happily. Some examples for me would be cottage cheese, melon balls, or a slice of crustless vegetable quiche.

• Cheese is a compact energy food that I prefer to eat by itself for the taste, and not disguised in a dish. I usually grate mozzarella and keep it handy in the refrigerator, since it's one of the lowest-calorie cheeses (80 per ounce) and it's tasty to me when I crave a cheese snack.

• Cantaloupe is one of the best foods you can have around the house. A half cup of these melon balls contains only 30 calories, making them ideal for breakfast, snacks or as an appetizer before dinner. Cantaloupe also provides more Vitamin A *per calorie* than any other fruit and contains as much Vitamin C *per calorie* as most citrus fruits.

• When snacking, eat orange and grapefruit *slices* instead of drinking them as juice. You'll feel more as if you've eaten something, and it takes longer, so you'll be less tempted to find something else to eat.

• I once was a potato-chip junkie, eating them at will two or three times a week. I knew they were deadly to any sane eating plan (10 chips have 115 calories—and who can stop at 10 chips?), but I didn't cut back until I learned that when a whole potato is converted to eight ounces of potato chips, the chef adds 28 teaspoons of shortening. At 37 calories per teaspoon, that's approximately 1,000 calories used to create a small bag of chips, not to mention all that fat. Can you believe it! So why not have a baked potato (about 140 calories) and at least *see* the calories you add with butter? (Of course, potato chips are not the only culprits; the same could basically be said about corn chips and peanuts.)

• Shelled almonds represent a more subtle trap. Although they're good for you nutritionally, they also have 425 calories in half a cup. This means they've become a *rare* taste treat for me, and even then I eat only two or three when I'm tempted.

• If possible, brush your teeth immediately after you finish lunch and dinner —before automatically treating yourself to a dessert. This cuts down your urge to snack soon afterwards, when your teeth are squeaky clean.

MAKING YOUR NEW EATING PLAN WORK

Since I believe in the joy of eating, it saddens me when I hear somebody complain, "I can't eat that—I'm on a diet." That feeling of deprivation is one important reason why I oppose the "dieting" concept for losing weight or keeping one's weight in check. If you're trying to be faithful to a strict diet and continually have to deny yourself little eating pleasures, then you're not living each day to the fullest. And, if you're continually "cheating" on your diet, the resulting guilt can easily lead to more binges.

Although I rigorously control my weight, I always leave room for desirable eating opportunities that might arise. For instance, if I want to be extra trim for a photography session or television appearance, I'm *better* about what I eat the week beforehand; I cut back and cut down in little ways—and I never let up with my daily aerobic exercising. Yet if I'm invited out to dinner at a fabulous restaurant, then I'd be sacrificing too much pleasure if I said, "I can't go, I'm cutting down this week." I go and enjoy myself, eating modestly but savoring the whole experience of being there.

Controlling your weight will always require continual juggling, determination, and a flexible attitude. An overall eating plan for the week ahead is important, but so is having the confidence to adapt to the unexpected. If relatives or close friends come into town, you should be able to enjoy entertaining them with pleasurable meals. You may blow your eating plan for a particular day, but you can minimize the damage by getting an aerobic workout and compensating the next day or later in the week. (If you have guests for two weeks, well . . . haul out your extra reserves of willpower.)

When you start your campaign to change certain eating habits, beware of the saboteurs! Be proud of what you're doing for yourself and your body, but unless you have a supportive spouse or close friend, it might be wise not to tell anyone. Sad but true, some people don't want to see others succeeding at improving themselves, and they will subtly try to sabotage these efforts with snide remarks or tempting offers to indulge.

This was brought home to me by a dear friend who said, "When I'm

SIX FOR MOTIVATION

I hope you've found many new hints in this chapter that you can now quietly incorporate into your daily life. Whenever your willpower weakens, review this checklist:

1. It takes patience, honesty, and a positive approach to change ingrained habits. So be kind to yourself as you go along and have confidence that you *can* change your eating patterns.

2. You're trying to improve yourself gradually and painlessly, so don't try to be too good too soon. That usually leads to dropping out.

3. If you're aerobically fit and you want to lose weight—but can't seem to drop those pounds—then you must reexamine and readjust your eating habits until you're eating smarter in a way that's comfortable for you.

4. If you're still sedentary and unsuccessful in losing fat by cutting calories alone, then you should go back and read Chapter Three, "Whistle, Whistle, Let's Go!" Begin to open new doors, get out, and *move!*

5. If you're conscientious but you feel you're not losing weight as fast as you'd like, remember that a healthy weight-loss goal is one pound a week. That's over 50 pounds a year! To lose a pound a week, you only need to increase your physical activity and decrease your food intake by a combined total of 500 calories a day.

6. Determine how much weight you need to lose in order to feel good about yourself, then think in terms of weekly one-pound losses. Take bite-size steps and reward yourself with a non-eating treat as you achieve a particular goal. When you reach your destination, you'll have an eating plan that fits your lifestyle.

eating something I vowed I wasn't going to touch—then changed my mind —nothing upsets me more than to have someone, especially my husband, tell me: 'I thought you were on a diet! No wonder you're not losing weight.' I just want to say, 'It's none of your business,' but instead I take another helping because I'm mad and I'm hurt."

So, while you're working on an improved eating plan that you're confident you can follow, why take any extra chances by telling everyone? However, there's one person you should consult with before starting on any weight-reduction plan, and that's your doctor.

Take a positive approach when you're trimming your eating. Once you've made a commitment, remember that acquiring better habits is gradual and you should pride yourself in taking even the smallest steps. For example, why not try taking the skin off your chicken? If you're currently eating chicken in some form four times a week and you can manage to skin it twice a week, you're not giving up chicken skin—you're just modifying your intake. Pretty soon you'll very likely discover that you're no longer eating chicken skin at all.

Gradually lead yourself down the garden path. Instead of thinking that you're giving up favorite taste treats, open yourself up to *new* tastes that will make you feel good about yourself. I've learned to tell myself, "I like all kinds of food, but I'm going to learn to prefer the foods that are better for me—nutritionally and calorie-wise—and I'm going to phase out the foods I really shouldn't eat, except as an occasional treat." This is the way new habits happen!

7

Safe and Sane Participation

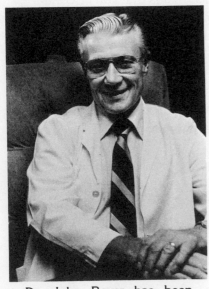

Dr. John Boyer has been medical director of the Exercise Physiology Laboratory and Adult Fitness Center at San Diego State University since 1965.

I first met Dr. John Boyer in 1974 when I attended an Adult Fitness Workshop in San Diego. I was so impressed with his knowledge in the area of physical fitness, as well as his personal dedication to fitness as a way of life, that I asked him if he would serve as my medical consultant. Happily, he agreed, and over the years I've asked him many questions relating to Aerobic Dancing so that we could always be assured of offering a safe, sound, and effective program.

When deciding on the topics to cover in a "lifestyle" book, I knew that important health and safety guidelines should be included. I compiled a list of questions covering the common areas of concern to anyone pursuing an active life, and Dr. Boyer agreed to let me interview him. So here's our own little "talk show."

JACKI: When we first met, you were an avid runner. Now you've cut back on your running. Was this because you were injured or was this for injury prevention?

DR. BOYER: Our bodies change as we get older and we can't always continue to do the same things. At least not as much as we used to do. Running is hard on ankles, knees, and the lower back, so to prevent problems in these areas I cut back on the number of miles I was running every week (from 30 to 12) and added stationary cycling, walking, and a mini-trampoline as exercise variations.

JACKI: So, in addition to the mental change-of-pace provided by a variety of fitness and sports activities, there are physical benefits as well?

DR. BOYER: Absolutely. Reducing the number of weight-bearing activities and substituting some that are non—weight-bearing helps in injury prevention.

JACKI: You taught me the phrase, "Get fit to play," and it has been one of your basic themes over the years. Could you elaborate a bit?

DR. BOYER: Sure. If you're physically fit when you take up a new sport or return to a seasonal favorite, you're going to be much less prone to injury because your body can handle the challenge. Fitness also gives you endurance, so you'll be able to put more into your sport and get more out of its challenges. This is going to make your sport more fun and that's going to motivate you to play more often. In addition, aerobic fitness increases your enjoyment of seasonal sports. For example, I receive letters from people who say, "I'm a better snow skier now because I have more endurance and I'm stronger. That means I don't have to spend the first week of vacation shaping up on the slopes; I'm in shape when I arrive and I can enjoy skiing from the first day on. And I'm not nearly as sore the next morning as I used to be."

JACKI: Everyone knows that exercising burns calories, but few people seem to know about the *after-exercise* bonus.

DR. BOYER: This bonus is exactly that, even though it isn't talked about a lot. It's a fact that it takes your body about four hours for its metabolic rate to return to what it was *before* your workout. This means that you're continuing to burn calories at a higher level during all those hours. So, you're burning calories while you're exercising, and bonus calories afterwards.

JACKI: It would seem then that breaking a one-hour workout into two half-hour workouts, one in the morning and one in the afternoon, would help burn more calories?

DR. BOYER: That's right. But 60 minutes of *continuous* exercise is more beneficial to your cardiovascular system (heart, lungs, and arteries) than two 30-minute workouts.

JACKI: Whenever possible, I try to exercise for one hour in the morning with a weight-bearing activity and one hour in the afternoon with a non—weight-bearing activity. That way I get both the calorie and aerobic benefits.

JACKI: You mentioned that as we get older our bodies change. We also seem to get a little heavier, don't we?

DR. BOYER: Yes, and there's an insidious process at work here. Once we pass age thirty-five, our basal metabolism slows down by two to five percent a year. That means that our body needs less fuel even at rest. If we don't either eat less or exercise a little more each year, we're going to store more fat.

JACKI: That's one of the main reasons I sit down on my birthday—*after* I've had my piece of cake—and plan how to add action and better eating choices to the upcoming year. It's a new *year's* resolution.

JACKI: I'm frequently asked about Aerobic Dancing, running, or doing any vigorous exercises during pregnancy. What about that?

DR. BOYER: Every woman should check with her physician, but generally, if she has been active before her pregnancy, there's no reason she shouldn't be able to continue at least through the second trimester. In fact, it's beneficial to both the mother and the child.

JACKI: Pregnant students often tell me that it's easier to combat gaining too much weight by staying in my course as long as possible *and* they don't feel as ungainly when they move smoothly and gracefully at least two times a week (at a walking level, of course). As one woman wrote me, "I go to class and I fantasize . . . I'm gliding and even though I'm walking, I feel light as a feather for two hours a week."

JACKI: Some people put a lot of emphasis on how to breathe during exercise. Is there anything we should be especially aware of in this regard?

DR. BOYER: Breathing is a natural function, and one should remember to breathe in a normal, relaxed manner while exercising. What *is* dangerous is NOT breathing. Holding your breath—or just forgetting to breathe—decreases the return of carbon dioxide–laden blood to your lungs for the exchange of oxygen for your tissues. This can cause you to faint or at least to have to stop the exercise. A good tip to remember is, "Exhale on effort."

JACKI: A "rule of lungs" that I often recommend is you should be able to comfortably carry on a conversation with a companion (or yourself) when you're jogging or running—or, if you're in one of my classes, you should be able to shout out or sing along.

JACKI: As I travel around the country I'm amazed to still see runners (and even exercise leaders) vigorously *bouncing* while stretching.

DR. BOYER: So am I, because that's a good way to injure a muscle, ligament, or tendon. Most stretching should be done gently and statically, without bouncing. It's very easy to exceed the elastic capability of a muscle, ligament, or tendon, especially if they aren't warmed up properly, or haven't been stretched for some time. This is particularly true for hamstring, calf and back muscles. I would point out, however, that side-bend stretches can be done rhythmically.

JACKI: It's common knowledge that stretching increases flexibility, but how important is that flexibility to the aerobically active person?

DR. BOYER: From an injury prevention standpoint, it's very important. A lack of flexibility and failure to stretch properly before an exercise session or sport is just asking for an injury.

JACKI: That's why I'm so adamant about proper warm-up in my classes and in the Everyday Eights. Also, I can't stress enough how important calf stretches are at the *end* of vigorous workouts. However, not all stretches are safe for most people, are they?

DR. BOYER: That's true. Stretches that bring the fingers and toes together with the knees locked (for example, toe touches and straight-leg sit-ups) can potentially damage ligaments and discs in the back. Also, lying on your back on the floor and raising your legs back over your head until your toes touch the floor can injure your neck *and* back at the same time. And finally, many people have injured themselves by lying face down on the floor and arching their back by raising both arms and both legs off the floor at the same time.

JACKI: One of the ways we've kept our program safe is by always reminding our students to "dance tall," which simply means with good posture and proper body alignment. This helps prevent injuries like shinsplints. Why don't you explain just what shinsplits are?

DR. BOYER: The term is a catch-all for all tissue inflammation that occurs in the front of the lower leg. It is a deep-seated, throbbing pain, usually worse at night, and not relieved by much of anything except rest. It is most commonly caused by mechanical stresses transmitted to the small muscles attached to the tibia (the "shin bone").

JACKI: Will you tell us how shinsplints can be prevented?

DR. BOYER: The most important preventive measure is to analyze the running or dancing form and correct any mechanical problem (such as running with the feet pointed outward, or running by landing on the toes).

JACKI: Achilles' tendinitis also seems to be a common complaint, especially among runners and joggers. Just what is tendinitis and how can it be prevented?

DR. BOYER: This is a swollen, tender and disabling condition affecting the Achilles' tendon, located just above the heel. The condition often appears suddenly with no explanation. The tendon inflammation must be allowed to subside completely before restarting exercises.

JACKI: What if I'm not real careful and develop tendinitis? What should I do to treat it?

DR. BOYER: Rest the injured area, apply ice two to three times daily for several days, elevate the limb, and take aspirin to relieve the pain and the inflammation.

JACKI: What if, in spite of being cautious, you injure a muscle or joint? Not a break or anything serious—it just hurts. What's the best method of immediate treatment, ice or heat?

DR. BOYER: The preferred treatment is ice. It should be applied in a towel or plastic bag and should be kept moving to avoid frostbite of the area. Apply it for thirty minutes two to three times daily for a day or so.

JACKI: When I've had an injury or even minor aches and pains, I simply remember that "ice" stands for

Ice,
Compression (with a dash of compassion), and
Elevation.

I put an ice-filled cloth napkin around my foot or ankle, elevate my leg on a pillow on the couch, and read a good book on injury prevention.

JACKI: In many parts of the country, an active person is going to be forced to exercise outdoors in hot, humid weather at certain times of the year. What precautions do you recommend?

DR. BOYER: I think we should emphasize the warning that overheating and exercising in weather like this can certainly produce additional stress. Also, even in hot humid climates, the body's primary need is for fluids, not salt. Most people *never* need to consume extra salt after a hard workout, and nobody should ever, under any circumstances, use salt tablets. By the same token, you should always drink water if you're thirsty while exercising or afterwards, no matter what the weather.

JACKI: When it comes to injury prevention, exercise leaders often tell us, "Listen to your body." Could you elaborate on this advice?

DR. BOYER: Everybody should respect the onset of pain as the body's warning sign. They should discontinue exercise when pain is present, allow the area to rest, apply ice if necessary, and obtain medical attention if these home remedies do not stop the problem.

JACKI: Injuries can depress any of us. I've discovered from personal experience that the best thing to do when I'm injured is *some* kind of exercise —not only to promote healing, but to keep my spirits up.

DR. BOYER: That's the right approach, since complete rest when injured can cause a multitude of undesirable results:

- Stiffness in joints, ligaments, muscles, and tendons, which leads to decreased flexibility,
- Softening of the bones (they become harder when the body is active and under stress),
- Poor circulation and loss of blood vessel tone,
- Decrease in muscle size and strength,
- Decrease in pain tolerance, and
- Gradual decrease in aerobic fitness.

JACKI: How depressing! That's why I'm urging people to at least do the Everyday Eights and stationary cycling, swimming, or walking when they can't dance or jog. I also consider myself an athlete, and I know one of the most important messages we can give to any person who is addicted to movement is this reminder: When you're injured you become frustrated and the overwhelming tendency is to try to resume your sport too soon. Instead, you must give your injury the time it needs to completely heal, or you're just asking for greater troubles. Another doctor once told me, "It's not medicine that you need, Jacki, but a tincture of time."

DR. BOYER: I certainly would agree. The injured athlete at any level of involvement must treasure *patience* and respect the time necessary for any injury to heal properly.

JACKI: In Aerobic Dancing we usually have a two-week holiday break at the end of every year and we caution our students to take it easy when they start up again in January. What advice do you give your patients when they re-enter an exercise program after a layoff?

DR. BOYER: I stress moderation on re-entry to a fitness program. This is crucial. Begin, as you say, "at a walking level" and gradually return to the level of fitness you enjoyed before your layoff.

JACKI: I'd like to emphasize this by saying that "too much, too soon, too fast" usually equals aches and pains and frowns.

One more question about layoffs. What's the "hard/easy principle," and how does it affect us aerobic lifestylers?

DR. BOYER: When returning to any running or jumping activity, you should follow the hard/easy principle: after exercising legs and feet, give them a day of rest before running again. The reason for this is that the bones, ligaments, muscles, and joints will take time to regain their strength and must be given a day off to recover. An "easy" day can be some non–weight-bearing activity like swimming or stationary cycling.

JACKI: What about walking as a re-entry program?

DR. BOYER: Walking is an excellent way to get back into distance running, or to maintain a degree of fitness when you're forced to lay off your regular program for whatever reason. I would also reiterate, Jacki, that walking in and of itself is a terrific activity for millions of people, not just those who are injured.

JACKI: Thousands of exercise facilities have opened in recent years, and many of them feature exercise machines. Not all of these machines are effective, are they?

DR. BOYER: That's right. Only the machines that make you work are effective. Treadmills, stationary bicycles and resistance machines are in this category because you are active. Machines that roll, pound, or shake you are called "passive" machines and they do nothing for you.

JACKI: Another item in this category is rubber or plastic exercise suits. Every time I see people running in one of these suits I want to stop and tell them how potentially dangerous they are.

DR. BOYER: You'd be doing them a favor, Jacki. These suits aren't effective because all of the weight loss they cause is due to water loss. And they're dangerous because they don't allow perspiration to evaporate for proper body cooling. This can drive the body temperature up to dangerous levels.

JACKI: We ought to also include the rubber belts that people wear around their waist to lose inches off their waistline—which causes nothing but water loss, too. They're called sauna belts and I see ads for them in practically every health and fitness magazine.

Since this is turning into a "heated" discussion, let's remind readers that hot tubs, saunas, steam rooms, Jacuzzis and whirlpools fail to provide any fitness benefits.

DR. BOYER: Right, and they are potentially dangerous for individuals with high blood pressure and those on certain medications. However, this isn't to deny their benefits, since they're helpful for relaxation, for cleansing your pores, and are sometimes used for physical therapy as part of the injury-healing process. We should also reiterate our warning about the potential dangers of becoming dehydrated in saunas, steam rooms, and hot tubs.

JACKI: We hear a lot these days about working isolated muscles to exhaustion; that is, until they quiver or "burn." Is that a good practice?

DR. BOYER: It's not particularly dangerous, but neither is it especially effective. The "burn" is caused by waste products building up in the muscle faster than the bloodstream can carry them away. This is working the muscle to excess. It would be better to do a comfortable number of repetitions, then give the bloodstream the time to do its job—and then work that muscle again.

JACKI: It's easy to see that I was one of your students when you look at my Aerobic Dancing patterns. My theory has always been that it's just as effective and much more pleasurable to spread out the repetitions and avoid that exercise-to-excess feeling.

One of the pieces of misinformation that I find widespread concerns spot reducing. The myth bothers me because it can lead to frustration and maybe abandoning an exercise program. We have to tell people we don't lose fat only from the spot we are exercising. Fat is burned from all over the body, and you'll notice it disappearing first from the place where it was deposited last (which for most people is the face).

DR. BOYER: That's true. It's possible to do spot *exercises* which will work on isolated muscles, but spot *reducing* is simply not possible. Instead of trying to attack fat in this manner, people should turn to aerobic exercises. These are the high-calorie burners and they melt fat faster from all over the body.

JACKI: I believe that the reason this false belief in spot reducing is perpetuated is the hope people have of dealing with cellulite.

DR. BOYER: I'm glad you brought this up. For, as you know, cellulite is a fiction. It simply does not exist as a separate type of fat that must be dealt with any differently. Understandably, women want attractive legs, and unfortunately this area is susceptible to the dimples of fat that people *call* cellulite. But the fact remains: fat is fat and is not burned by the body from specific places. Instead, the only thing that will help is regular aerobic exercise and a healthy diet.

JACKI: I've always required that my instructors be physically fit role models for our students. Part of this image is a lean body weight which we measure with scales. I know that caliper measurements or hydrostatic weighing are more accurate, but can't most people rely on scales?

DR. BOYER: In most cases, the balance scale or bathroom scale provides a good measure of body fat. Better yet, people ought to simply look at themselves in the mirror. The other methods may be more accurate, but are not practical for most individuals or available on a widespread basis. They are tools of the laboratory where a greater degree of accuracy is required by researchers.

JACKI: One last question. I'm often asked if exercise will help us live longer. Since any one of us could have an accident at any time, I emphasize the *quality* of life that comes with regular exercise. What do you say?

DR. BOYER: There is no concrete evidence that exercise will increase life expectancy or prevent certain diseases such as a heart attack. However, exercise, good nutrition, maintaining proper weight, stopping smoking (or better yet, not starting), learning to handle stress, and having a positive mental outlook all contribute to better energy and stamina—and more joy in our life for whatever number of years we have left.

JACKI: That's what the aerobic lifestyle is all about. The quality of life! And of course you know I have special lyrics for this thought:

> *Thunderclouds have their lightning,*
> *Nightingales have their song,*
> *Don't you see we want our lives*
> *to be something more than long?*

8

There's No Stopping You Now!

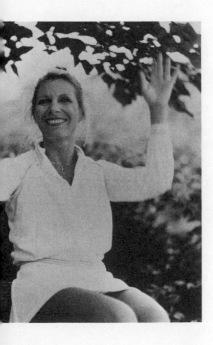

My ultimate goal in the aerobic lifestyle is to join body and mind in a celebration of being alive. Toward that end, these are themes that I believe in and live by that help me tackle the challenges of life.

- Reach out, be open, and try to accept everyone.
- Welcome change . . . without it life is a bore.
- Approach challenges one step at a time.
- Gently and progressively grow and be better.
- Optimism . . . hope . . . LOVE.
- Be spontaneous.
- Play . . . PRETEND.
- Don't take yourself too seriously.
- Live each day . . . really LIVE it!

One of the most motivating experiences I've ever had was reading Leo Buscaglia's best seller, *Living, Loving & Learning.* His theme and the way he reaches out and hugs life lifted my spirits, because his philosophy is so close to what I've been trying to express through Aerobic Dancing. He urges us to live each day to the fullest—or, as he puts it, "Look at things for the first time with the wonder of a child." And I loved it when he said, "When you hear yourself saying, 'I'm too old for that,' you're also closing doors. You're never too old for anything! Because age is in your head, nowhere else."

Leo inspired me, and I hope I've inspired you—in my own way—to set new goals and to start making the little changes in your life that add up to important changes. In fact, why not think of this book as a sabbatical? You've discovered some new facts, ideas, and insights, but how are you going to use this information? What directions will you take to experience new "healthy highs" in your daily life? Don't cheat yourself by doing nothing. I've given you some hints and helpful guidelines on how you can live life more aerobically. So now it's time for *you* to set up some do-able goals.

You're ready to take a different direction in your approach to eating, exercise, and living life. But first take the time to get a perspective on what you've read and how it relates to what you've been doing and what you're going to do. You may look at your situation and think, "I need six months to do that, but I can only squeeze out one day." Fine! Just make the most of the time you have, and don't sit around daydreaming . . . make concrete plans.

LIVING YOUR DREAMS

I've always believed in thinking and dreaming big, and so I readily identify with Barry Manilow's song, "Riders to the Stars." The lyrics say it perfectly:

> *The dreamer dreams on, and*
> *dreams never die,*
> *as long as we try.*
> *Gotta believe!*
> *Gotta reach out!*

So many people are afraid to risk failure or rejection in any aspect of life, whether it means trying to expand and make new friends, learning a sport, or creating a new challenge in their business. Their motto is "Better safe than sorry." My motto is "No risk, no rapture."

The biggest dream I've had in my life was a nationwide Danceathon in November 1981, to raise money for the Special Olympics. Our goal was to raise millions of dollars in pledges tied to how many dances my students could do in four-hour danceathons to be held in 117 cities over one weekend. It took the philosophy I'm sharing in this book to make this happening happen.

Like Pac-Man eating an entire maze of dots, one dot at a time, we took on this enormous project one step at a time. I convinced my national staff that it was a great idea, and then gave them binders that said, "How to Dance-a-Thon" . . . except that the binders were empty. I didn't want to overwhelm them, so we sent them one "chapter" at a time, every few weeks. As they reached each new step of the procedure, they received the information they needed.

Meanwhile, I was traveling the country saying we were going to raise millions of dollars, and my friends told me later they were fearful—for me—because they were afraid I was going to be proved wrong. But I wasn't worried; I was excited. We were working for the Special Olympics, a group close to our hearts, and I knew all we had to do was persuade our students to keep dancing for four hours. Their overwhelming response was to "dance the distance"—a total of fifty dances! After doing this, they felt terrific about themselves; they felt like athletes. They then took their aerobic bodies out into the winter cold and collected their pledges. And guess what? They were so proud, and their friends and neighbors were so amazed at what they had accomplished, that more money was donated than was originally pledged. This was the magic part of the whole event—a dream come true! We raised over four million dollars in two days. *So don't be afraid to dream!*

> Got a dream, boy.
> Got a song.
> Paint your wagon and come along!

Now I have another dream for the eighties. I want to make fitness as popular as cigarettes and liquor. I'm going to do it, and you can help.

Have you ever seen a liquor advertisement that said, "Drink, because if you don't, you'll feel nervous and self-conscious at social gatherings?" Have you ever seen a cigarette billboard that said, "Smoke, because if you don't you're liable to gain weight?" Of course you haven't. So why do people keep saying, "Exercise, because if you don't your muscles will sag"? Or, "Exercise, because if you don't you'll be more prone to fatigue." How negative!

We need a new positive approach, spotlighting the fact that fitness IS the good way of life. It IS the fun way of life. It IS the way to feel as youthful as the models on the cigarette and liquor billboards look. So focus your attention on the glamour of fitness and the thrill of physically participating. Just lose yourself in the happiness of having played the fitness game that day, that hour, that minute.

COPING WITH STRESS

I'm such an outspoken believer in optimism that you might be thinking, "Jacki, are you always this energized? Are you always this happy?" Well, I'll be honest: Of course there are times when I feel angry, deflated, or even defeated, and I realize I'm spending very precious time focusing on negative details when I should be allowing myself to see the big beautiful picture. Then there are days when I feel empty, usually after I've completed the choreography for a session, or following a cross-country trip when jet lag catches me. This is emotional fatigue that results from the stress of responding to exciting experiences and creative projects. I know I'm susceptible to this kind of letdown and I try to remind myself that all it takes is a little rest, a little relaxation, and a change of pace. Then, sure enough, I wake up and have all my optimism back to meet new challenges with enthusiasm.

I know that all of you who are physically fit are going to be active in *many* ways. You're most likely juggling lots of things in life and still finding the time you need to keep in shape. However, there will be those "down" days when nothing goes right and one commitment after another steals the time you treasure for yourself. At times like this, consider some of the ways I've learned to handle stress:

1. Every day has its unique challenges, but the going is easier if you can step back and laugh at yourself or the situation you're in. I once choreographed a cool-down dance to "I Made it Through the Rain," and in my notes to students I said, "I try to think that every shower makes us grow a bit . . . The real secret is to keep your sense of humor, because there's always the chance you'll hear laughter in the rain." So why not *practice* seeing the good in everything that happens?

2. When somebody asks, "How do you balance all the things in your life? my answer is, "I don't." I can't balance every day or even every week in an organized way, but I have a challenging life that makes me happy because I know that all the different facets are getting the attention they deserve: Neil, Aerobic Dancing, my family and friends, and my personal fitness. I approach it like a circus performer who keeps all the plates spinning on their sticks. When I see one plate start to slow down and begin to fall, I race over and get it going again, and then I run to another plate and get it going as it wobbles. If it falls—well, we all make mistakes, we're only human—I pick it up and get it going again.

3. Don't always try to contain yourself—it's too safe. It's also healthier to experience all emotions, learn from them, and accept them. If you were happy ALL the time, "happy" would mean nothing. There'd be no value to "happy" because there would be nothing to compare it to. Remember in Chapter One when I told you that a fitness workout will give you more energy by burning off excess adrenaline? Well, researchers now say—and I know it's true from personal experience—that it's good mental, emotional, and even physical therapy to let yourself go: release your feelings, whether they be of anger, fear, frustration, laughter, or joy. If you're one of my students and these emotions come out in class, great! In fact, laughing and crying can increase the hemoglobin in your blood, which in turn helps make you feel better.

4. Obviously, you can't take all the stress out of your life, and you wouldn't want to, because then you'd be bored. But you can start to examine your stress and say, "I can't get a handle on all of this at once, but there are a few little things I can do." Change some of your everyday patterns so you can let off steam and have a little less pressure on yourself. Pick one area and focus on it. For example, if you get cramps in your shoulder because you sit at your desk for three hours at a stretch, change just that one aspect of your day. Get up and walk around the office for five minutes every hour, and do the first six movements from the Everyday Eights. It's that easy!

5. Learn to be resilient. When something goes wrong and your initial instinct is to think, Well, there's just nothing I can do about that situation, try to say, "Hold it! There must be a choice here. I need to look for another option."

6. Having a pet or an aquarium is a fun, loving way to help relieve stress. Just taking time out to do something as simple as stroking your pet is good for your blood pressure, besides being good for the pet. Holding and hugging my cats are daily pleasures. I'll sit down in my studio for hours working on a project and our cats, Rowdy and Elliott, will sometimes both be in my lap. I love it. Their purring is very calming as I work.

TAKE TIME OUT TO LIVE EACH DAY

My fellow aerobic lifestyler, George Sheehan, said it so well: "Living now is life itself!" Sure it's great to be an adult, but to really *enjoy* living a multifaceted life, make sure you take time out each day to relax and take yourself a little less seriously. Or, as a friend put it, "Who said we have to be full-time adults? I like to be a part-time adult."

I get a warm feeling every time I read the lyrics to "Smile, Smile, Smile." They remind me how important it is to treasure all the beautiful little moments in life:

> *I saw a sparkle of rain*
> *I saw a kiss in a rose . . .*
> *I felt a butterfly's wings*
> *I felt it tickle my nose*
> *It made me smile, smile, smile.*
>
> *I heard the whole world sing*
> *And bells start to chime*
> *The day a baby walked*
> *For the very first time!*
>
> *The smallest moment of joy*
> *Can fill your heart with a smile*
> *And make it all worth while!*
>
> *Hey, what's that look on your face*
> *The world's a much better place*
> *I saw you smile, smile, SMILE!*

LET YOUR PLAYFUL SIDE EMERGE

Leo Buscaglia wrote, "If you become alive by dancing through the world, swinging from the trees, doing kooky things, you become and stay exciting." Or, as I would say . . .

—Do a "summer"sault, fallsault, wintersault, or a springsault!
—Surprise people.
—Hide.
—Laugh so hard you cry.

—Cry so hard you laugh at what a sorry sight you are.

—Chase a butterfly, not to catch it but to get to see its beauty longer.

—Pour a glass of water over your head after a fitness workout . . . or run through the sprinklers! When I run at my dad's ranch in Florida, it's heaven to douse myself with a hose.

In other words, be more childlike. When I'm asked, "Do people ever get too old for your program?" my answer is, "You're only too old for Aerobic Dancing if you're too old to pretend and play." If you're one of my students, then you know I feel it's okay for adults to pretend they're playing the guitar, dealing cards, snapping pictures with an imaginary camera, or dancing in a Broadway chorus line. Some of my students have to be led down the road to being a child again, but once our instructors overcome their resistance, they become enthusiastic supporters. One woman, married to a corporation president, confided a typical feeling when she told me, "My husband would die if he saw the way I act up in class. But this is what I need. I love to hoot and holler and sing. I play and let myself go."

Personally, I love the idea of acting like a kid again, whether it's pretending, doing something goofy just because it looks like fun, or laughing out loud at some crazy happening or a funny friend. And it doesn't matter if I'm alone or with other people; my playful side can emerge at almost any time. Maybe this attitude seems a bit frivolous for a woman who celebrated forty action-packed years in 1982, but this is the aerobic lifestyle spirit!

SHARING AND CARING

I want to share what I can give.
I want to be,
I want to live!

When Aerobic Dancers meet me for the first time, they say it's like seeing a long-lost friend. They feel they know me very well because of the way I have opened up through my dances. Now that you and I have spent a few hours together—me talking and you listening (and I hope sometimes talking back or at least shouting in agreement), I'm feeling as I did when I ended my first book with the words, "Have fun, keep fit." That made me a little sad, because I knew I would never meet most of my at-home Aerobic Dancers in person.

I have that same feeling again, because I know I can't shake your hand right now, or give you a hug. But I feel like we're fitness friends because I've been sharing my dreams and ideas with you, and that's what friendship is all about. I care about you, and I know you're going to have many success stories living the aerobic lifestyle. So come on, share these stories with me. I'd love to hear from you. And remember: THERE'S NO STOPPING YOU NOW!

Jacki's Theme: "There's No Stopping Us!"

There's no stoppin' us
We ain't had enough
We won't quit till we stand up
Turn on the world
With what we've done
There's more to come
Every move that we make
Brings us closer to
Turnin' on the world
There's no stoppin' us
We ain't had enough
We're a team and we're gonna make it
We ain't had enough
There's no stoppin' us
Look out world, we're a team

We ain't sittin' back
Life's too short for that
We're all winners each time we go out and try
Like we said, there's so much ahead
Every step that we take
Brings us closer to being the winners we are
A-E-R-O-B-I-C-S . . . Let's Go!

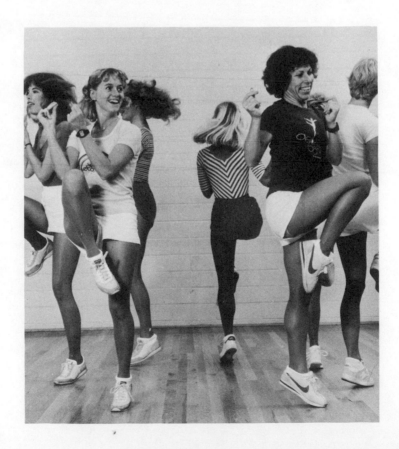

ABOUT THE AUTHORS

Jacki Sorensen, the originator of Aerobic Dancing, is one of the best-known figures in the American fitness field. She is a consultant to the President's Council on Physical Fitness and Sports, and in 1982 she was awarded the National Honor Award from the Council. Jacki, a professional dancer, choreographer, and lecturer, travels extensively while directing the activities of Aerobic Dancing, Inc., which offers her unique program throughout the U.S.A. and overseas. Jacki and her husband, Neil, live in Malibu, California.

Bill Bruns, sports editor at *Life* magazine until 1972, is the co-author of nine books in the fitness field, including Vic Braden's *Tennis for the Future* and, with Jacki Sorensen, *Aerobic Dancing.* He lives with his wife, Pam, and their two children, Alan and Allison, in Pacific Palisades, California.